New technologies in the fight against transboundary animal diseases

FAO
ANIMAL
PRODUCTION
AND HEALTH
PAPER
144

FAO-Japan Cooperative Project:
Collection of Information on Animal Production and Health
Phase One: Transbounday Animal Diseases

EMPRES
EMERGENCY PREVENTION SYSTEM

Food
and
Agriculture
Organization
of
the
United
Nations

FIAT PANIS

Rome, 1999

M-27
ISBN 92-5-104358-2

ACKNOWLEDGEMENT

This report is a product of the FAO-Japan Cooperative Project 'Collection of Information on Animal Production and Health', with support of the Japan Racing Association (JRA) fund.

It has been prepared by Drs. Chris Baldock, Tony Forman, Bill Geering and Bill Taylor, in collaboration with the Infectious Diseases-EMPRES Group, Animal Health Service, Animal Production and Health Division, FAO

ACKNOWLEDGEMENTS

[illegible]

[illegible]

Contents

Acronyms used in the Text

ASF	African swine fever
BSE	Bovine spongiform encephalopathy
CBPP	Contagious bovine pleuropneumonia
CFT	Complement fixation test
CSF	Classical swine fever
CJD	Creutzfeld Jakob Disease
DNA	Deoxyribose nucleic acid
ELISA	Enzyme linked immunosorbent assay
FAO	Food and Agriculture Organisation
FMD	Foot-and-mouth disease
GIS	Geographical information system
GPS	Geographical positioning system
IAEA	International Atomic Energy Agency
ISCOM	Immune stimulating complex
LSD	Lumpy skin disease
MAb	Monoclonal antibody
MHC	Major histocombatability complex
PARC	Pan African Rinderpest Campaign
PCR	Polymerase chain reaction
PPR	Peste des Petits Ruminants
RNA	Ribose nucleic acid
RP	Rinderpest
RT/PCR	Reverse Transcriptase Polymerase Chain Reaction
RVF	Rift Valley fever
TSE	Transmissable spongiform encephalopathies
WHO	World Health Organisation
VN	Virus neutralisation

Chapter 1

Transboundary Animal Diseases

1.1 Nature and potential consequences of transboundary animal diseases

All animal diseases have the potential to adversely affect human populations by reducing the quantity and/or quality of food, other livestock products (hides, skins, fibers) and animal power (traction, transport) that can be obtained from a given quantity of resources and by reducing peoples' assets. Of these, transboundary animal diseases tend have the most serious consequences.

Transboundary animal diseases may be defined as those epidemic diseases which are highly contagious or transmissible and have the potential for very rapid spread, irrespective of national borders, causing serious socio-economic and possibly public health consequences. These are diseases which cause a high morbidity and mortality in susceptible animal populations and they constitute a constant threat to the livelihood of livestock farmers. Furthermore, their potential consequences are of such a magnitude that their occurrence may also have a significant detrimental effect on national economies.

Transboundary animal diseases have the potential to:

- threaten food security through serious loss of animal protein and/or loss of draught animal power for cropping;
- increase poverty levels particularly in poor communities that have a high dependence on livestock farming for sustenance;
- cause major production losses for livestock products such as meat; milk and other dairy products; wool and other fibres and skins and hides, thereby reducing farm incomes. They may also restrict opportunities for upgrading the production potential of local livestock industries by making it difficult to utilise exotic high producing breeds which tend to be very susceptible to the transboundary diseases;
- add significantly to the cost of livestock production through the necessity to apply costly disease control measures;
- seriously disrupt or inhibit trade in livestock and livestock products either within a country or internationally. Their occurrence may thereby cause major losses in national export income in significant livestock-producing countries;
- cause public health consequences in the case of those transboundary animal diseases which can be transmitted to humans (i.e. zoonoses);
- cause environmental consequences through die-offs in wildlife populations in some cases, and
- cause pain and suffering for affected animals.

Examples of the Consequences of Transboundary Animal Diseases

Foot and mouth disease (FMD). In 1997 the disease seriously affected the commercial pig industry in Taiwan province of China, where 4 million pigs were slaughtered in order to control the epidemic.

Rinderpest. When this virus disease was first introduced to Africa in the late nineteenth century, it spread over almost the whole continent within 10 years, killing an estimated 10 million cattle and untold numbers of wildlife –irrevocably changing livestock husbandry and wildlife ecology there. In 1994, rinderpest spread to previously long-time free, remote mountainous areas of northern Pakistan killing an estimated 40,000 cattle and yaks.

Rift Valley fever (RVF). The first recorded outbreak of RVF in Egypt in 1977 caused an estimated 200,000 human cases of the disease with some 600 deaths as well as large numbers of deaths and abortions in sheep and cattle and other livestock species. An outbreak of the disease in East Africa in 1997-8 not only caused livestock losses and human deaths but also very seriously disrupted the valuable livestock export trade to the Middle East.

Contagious bovine pleuropneumonia (CBPP) There has been catastrophic spread of CBPP in Africa over the last few years where it now affects some 27 countries and causes estimated losses of up to $2 billion annually. In 1995 the disease was re-introduced to Botswana for the first time in 46 years. As part of the eradication campaign, all cattle in an area of northern Botswana had to be slaughtered at a direct cost of $100 million, although indirect losses would have been much higher.

Hog Cholera (or classical swine fever). A recent serious outbreak of the disease in the Netherlands led to the death or slaughter of some 12 million pigs as part of the eradication campaign. The cost of the Dutch outbreaks was estimated to be $US 2.35 billion, half of which was public money. The effects of the epidemic were so severe that the Dutch government approved a national pig restructuring plan which foresaw a reduction in the national pig herd of about 25% within 2 years.

African swine fever occurred for the first time in Cote d'Ivoire in 1996, where it killed 25% of the pig population and cost the country according to various estimates between $US 13 and 32 million. It has since spread to other countries in the region including Nigeria.

Highly pathogenic avian influenza An economic analysis of outbreaks of HPAI in Pennsylvania, USA in 1983-4 showed that the direct costs of eradication were $US 64 million, and the indirect costs to consumers were $500 million through increased prices of products. On the other hand, it was estimated that HPAI would have cost the US poultry industry $US 2 billion annually if it had become endemic. The influenza virus causing an outbreak of HP AI in Hong Kong in 1997 was found to be capable of transfer to humans and as a consequence a decision was taken to completely depopulate the 1.4 million chickens there.

Transboundary animal diseases constitute only a small minority of the infectious diseases that afflict livestock. All of the infectious diseases cause some of the above adverse socio-economic consequences to a greater or lesser extent, and in fact the cumulative production and economic losses that they cause is probably much greater than that of the so called transboundary animal diseases. However, what sets the transboundary diseases apart is the suddenness, acuteness and widespread nature of the losses that they can produce.

Another important characterising feature of transboundary animal diseases is the rapidity with which they can spread in susceptible livestock populations. This renders individual farmers and private veterinary services relatively powerless to take effective action to avoid or overcome outbreaks of these diseases. The responsibility for prevention, control and elimination of transboundary animal therefore falls squarely on the shoulders of the public sector, notably government veterinary services, .and may require high public investment. Furthermore these endeavours are only likely to be successful if government veterinary services are very well organised and prepared for these tasks.

As their name implies, transboundary animal diseases are no respectors of national or administrative borders. The control efforts of individual countries against these diseases may be continually frustrated by the fact that neighboring countries are not taking equivalent action. Transboundary animal diseases therefore need to be tackled on a regional basis, with cooperation between countries and harmonisation of their prevention and response programmes. An international approach also allows better advantage to be taken of natural geographical barriers and broader epidemiological patterns for the diseases.

1.2 Some major transboundary animal diseases and their current geographical distribution

Many transboundary animal diseases are caused by viruses. Important viral diseases include:

Foot-and-mouth disease(FMD): this is perhaps the most contagious disease of animals, affecting mainly cattle, sheep and pigs. Although not generally a killing disease it causes high morbidity and production losses, and is a major impediment to international trade in livestock and livestock products. The disease has been absent from south eastern Europe for over two years and from the rest of Europe for much longer. Considerable progress has been made towards eradication in South America, with the southern countries of Chile, Argentina, Paraquay, and Uruguay not having recorded outbreaks for two years or longer and the southern states of Santa Catarina and Rio Grande do Sul have been declared 'FMD free with vaccination'. FMD is still endemic in many parts of Africa, the Middle East and Asia, but a regional control programme is in place in South-East Asia.

Rinderpest (RP). This is a generalised virus disease affecting mainly cattle and buffaloes. It usually causes a very high mortality, although less virulent virus strains circulating in East Africa have complicated eradication there. RP has been progressively eliminated in West Africa, but here are still three endemic foci in East Africa. Great progress has been made towards RP eradication in India, but the disease is endemic in Pakistan and has spread to Afghanistan. There are endemic foci in the Middle. Sporadic outbreaks, the origins of which are unknown, have occurred in Eastern Russia and Mongolia in recent years.

Peste des petits ruminants (PPR) is a rinderpest-like disease of sheep and goats. In recent years there has been serious spread of this disease from Africa, to the Middle East and in Asia as far east as India.

Rift Valley Fever (RVF) is a serious mosquito-borne virus disease of sheep, cattle and goats which causes very high mortality rates in young animals and abortion of pregnant animals. It is also transmitted to humans causing a potentially fatal disease. Major epidemics have occurred at irregular intervals of 10-30 years in the eastern half of Africa, from South Africa to Egypt.
Lumpy skin disease (LSD) is a disease of cattle which may cause serious production losses, through prolonged debility and loss of hides. LSD is mainly confined to Africa, where it has caused periodic, major epidemics in many countries.

Classical swine fever (CSF) is a generalised virus disease of pigs which may cause high mortalities. It is endemic in much of South and South-East Asia , where it is a constraint to the development of the pig industry. It is the most significant transboundary animal disease in Europe, where it caused 611 outbreaks in the European Community in 1997. These occurred in the Netherlands, Germany, Spain and Italy and are estimated to have cost these countries more than $7 billion. Recent outbreaks have also occurred in Latin America.

African swine fever (ASF). is another generalised virus disease of pigs which is endemic in much of sub-Saharan Africa. There have been very serious outbreaks over the last few years in previously free areas of West Africa. ASF has shown great propensity for inter-continental spread an outbreaks have occurred at different times in parts of Europe and Latin America.

Newcastle disease (ND) is perhaps the most lethal disease of poultry, outbreaks of which have occurred in most parts of the world, including two major pandemics during this century. It is a major constraint to the development of village chicken industries, particularly in Asia and Africa.

Highly pathogenic avian influenza (HPAI) this is another serious poultry disease, which may produce high mortalities. There is some concern about the potential for the appearance of avian influenza virus strains transmittable to humans. Wild waterbirds constitute the major reservoir for avian influenza viruses and HPAI outbreaks in domestic poultry may occur suddenly anywhere in the world There have been a number of outbreaks in recent years in North America and Australia.

There is one important mycoplasmal transboundary animal disease. This is

Contagious bovine pleuropneumonia (CBPP). Although this is an insidious disease in areas where it is well established, it causes serious epidemics with high mortality rates in cattle when it moves into new areas. Major CBPP epidemics have been experienced in Eastern, Southern and West Africa over the last few years. The disease is also endemic in some parts of Asia.

1.3 Trends affecting transboundary animal diseases

Transboundary animal diseases exhibit a great deal of dynamism. New diseases emerge, and old diseases re-emerge. They show a great propensity for sudden and unexpected spread to new regions, often over great distances. These trends are likely to continue and even accelerate in the future.

The last 30 years or so have been remarkable for the emergence of apparently new infectious diseases. This has been spectacular in the medical field, with the appearance of diseases such as AIDS, Lassa fever, and Ebola. The same has occurred with animal diseases, with the appearance of bovine spongiform encephalopathy, porcine reproductive and respiratory syndrome (PRRS) and equine morbillivirus disease. Not only do new infections emerge, but also new biotypes or antigenic types of existing infectious diseases. A notable example has been the hypervirulent form of infectious bursal disease which has swept across much of Europe and Asia in recent years causing devastating losses to poultry industries there.

There are a number of factors contributing to the dynamic nature of transboundary animal diseases. These include:

- *increasing globalisation and international transport.* The most important method of spread of transboundary animal diseases is by movement of potentially infected livestock and meat and other animal products. There have been very substantial increases in such international movements due to better sea, land and air transport of people, animals and goods and in response to marketing opportunities for livestock and their products. Nomadism, transhumance, and the movement of refugees and their animals away from wars and civil disturbances also contribute very substantially to the spread of infectious animal diseases. These all place a great strain on countries in maintaining effective quarantine barriers at airports, seaports and along international borders;

- *changes in livestock production systems*. In many countries there is a trend towards increased intensification and commercialisation of livestock production particularly in peri-urban areas. The greater concentration of animals that this entails means that there is far greater opportunity for transboundary animal diseases to move very rapidly and for greater economic losses to occur;

- *decline in government veterinary services and other infrastructure*. Also in many countries public funding of veterinary services is poor and even declining, resulting in uncontrolled livestock movements, poor diagnostic capacity and the inability to react quickly and effectively to disease outbreaks. Farmers are usually not compensated for disease losses and thus often tend to sell still healthy-looking livestock to reduce their financial losses when a disease problem is occurring on their farm. As a proportion of these apparently healthy animals may be in early stages of infection where clinical signs are not yet apparent, this behavior of farmers may significantly contribute to the spread of disease;

- *spread of livestock farming into new ecosystems*. In some regions of the world, tropical rain forests and other wilderness areas are being converted to livestock farming. This places human communities and their farm animals into close contact with a completely new range of infectious diseases which may have previously only circulated in wild life reservoirs and which may be completely unknown. Some of these diseases may be transmittable to humans and/or livestock, in which they may spread very rapidly in the new, fully susceptible hosts;

- *global warming* trends may change rainfall and weather patterns in a number of regions, affecting particularly the global distribution of insect vectors, e.g. mosquitoes and *Culicoides* midges and the important viral and protozoal transboundary animal diseases that they transmit.

1.4 Combatting transboundary animal diseases

An effective national animal quarantine system should always be the first line of defence against the entry and establishment of transboundary animal diseases. However even the most sophisticated quarantine service cannot provide an absolute barrier. Countries therefore need a second line of defence , which is the development of contingency plans and capabilities to respond quickly to high threat diseases should they enter.

If an introduced transboundary animal disease can be recognised early whilst it is localised and then a disease control programme be quickly implimented, the prospects for eradication of the disease with minimal production losses and other costs are markedly enhanced. Conversely, if the disease is allowed to become well established in the country, eradication may be very costly and difficult or even impractical (particularly if the disease becomes established in wildlife).

Thus, the two key principles in combatting transboundary animal diseases are:

- **Early warning** . This is to rapidly detect the introduction of, or sudden increase in the incidence of any disease of livestock which has the potential of developing to epidemic proportions and/or causing serious socio-economic consequences or public health. concerns. It embraces all initiatives, mainly based on disease surveillance, reporting and epidemiological analysis that would lead to improved awareness and knowledge of the distribution and behaviour of disease outbreaks (and of infection) and which allow forecasting of the source and evolution of the disease outbreaks and the monitoring of the effectiveness of disease control campaigns, and

- **Early reaction.** This is is to carry out without delay the disease control activities needed to contain the outbreak and then to eliminate the disease and infection in the shortest possible time frame and in the most cost-effective way, or at least to return to the status-quo that which existed previously and to provide objective, scientific evidence that one of these objectives has been achieved.

1.5 The application of appropriate technology in the fight against transboundary animal diseases

The last twenty years or so have seen exceedingly rapid in scientific knowledge. This has been due in no small part to the revolution that has occurred in the fields of genetic engineering and computer science. Much new technology can now be applied to combat transboundary animal diseases. The areas in which technical advances to combat these diseases have been most pronounced are

- disease surveillance and animal health information systems
- other methods for studying the epidemiology of disease outbreaks
- disease diagnosis and methods for the characterisation of aetiological agents
- better vaccines for disease control and eradication programmes.

The aim of this report is to bring to the attention of professional workers in this field the newer technology that may be available to them in their endeavours against transboundary animal diseases.

All of the technology that will be described will not be appropriate for all countries or all circumstances. Indeed many of the more sophisticated techniques may only be suitable for specialist institutions such as International Reference Laboratories. It is important that an appropriate level of technology be selected for each situation, but that there should be a conscience effort on the part of national veterinary services to progressively improve their technical capabilities.

Chapter 2

ADVANCES IN EPIDEMIOLOGICAL AND ECONOMIC TECHNIQUES

2.1 Introduction

This chapter outlines some of the more important epidemiological and economic techniques relevant to reducing the risk of international spread of animal diseases as well as control of important epidemic diseases. These issues have always been the focus of international veterinary authorities. However, they have become even more important since the formation of the World Trade Organisation and subsequent implementation of the various multilateral agreements on trade. Consequent increased international trade in livestock commodities has resulted in increasing scrutiny of the risk of international spread of disease. As a result there has been a growing interest in developing better systems for investigating and reporting of animal diseases. For livestock, reliable evidence for freedom from particular diseases is becoming an issue of major interest. For this reason, the emphasis in this section is on animal health information systems and active disease surveillance programs.

2.2 Animal health information systems

An animal health information system is a system for the collection, storage, analysis and reporting of information related to the health of animals. As such, virtually every organised society that keeps animals has some form of animal health information system. This may range from the system used in a single village in a developing country (in which information is gathered by owners, passed by word of mouth, stored in the memory, analysed mentally, and further reported by word of mouth) to a national system such as that used in developed countries (involving a network of veterinary officers, laboratory diagnostic resources, complex sampling strategies, high powered computerised data management and analysis systems, and extensive procedures for distributing and acting upon the information gathered). This paper discusses larger scale animal health information systems, such as those used by national governments.

The word *system* implies a collection of many different components working together for a particular purpose. All too often, the expression *information system* gets mixed up with concepts of information technology, and is understood to refer to a computer system. Computers certainly play a role in most modern animal health information systems, but they are merely one component, a tool for handling the information. Instead, system here refers more to a set of operational and administrative procedures for the collection of data from a range of different sources, the processing of that data to produce useful information, and the application of that information to improve the well-being of animals and their owners.

The *animals* referred to may, of course, be any animals, although it is much more usual for a government run information system to deal with animals of perceived economic or social importance, primarily domestic animals. Information on farmed mammals, fish, crustaceans, and even insects (for instance bees) may be handled by such an information system, but the inclusion of data on wild animals is less common.

In general, the term *health* is used in a very broad sense. While information on the occurrence of animal diseases forms a large part of most systems, animal productivity information is often an important component. On the population level, health and productivity are very closely related and sometimes overlapping concepts.

The general structure of an animal information system and its relationships to data and decisions are shown in figure 1

Figure 1

The general structure of an animal information system

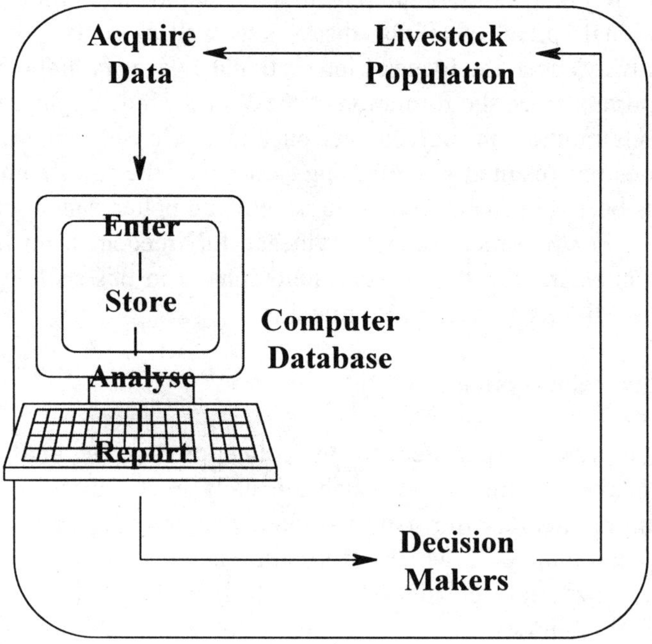

2.2.1 Objectives of an animal health information system

The objectives of an animal health information system vary according to the users of the information and the environment in which it is working. The overall objective is usually to provide information which enables decision makers to help improve or maintain the health and productivity of animals, and through this, the well-being of their owners and the wider community. This includes primarily information about the diseases present and their spatial distribution. A number of more specific objectives for an optimal system have been published (Morris, 1991; Thrusfield, 1995 p161; Martin *et al*, 1987 p260; Blajan, 1979; Blood and Brightling, 1988; Morley, 1988; Garner and Nunn, 1991; Martinez *et al*, 1992; Ellis, 1994). These can be grouped into four broad areas:

1. to collect basic animal health information
2. to help assess priorities and develop policies
3. to support the implementation of disease control programs
4. to meet international disease reporting obligations

These are further discussed below.

To collect basic animal health information. Basic animal health information is needed to identify what diseases are present, the level of the diseases, the distribution of the diseases, and the impact of the diseases.

The first requirement of any animal health information system is to identify the major animal health and production problems and their spatial distribution. Most systems in developed countries assume that this information is already well known. In developing countries, without a long history of animal health information collection, the government veterinary services may need to first collect basic information to determine which significant diseases are present in the country before addressing any of the other issues.

The next task is to obtain valid estimates of incidence and prevalence of the major disease problems. Quantitative estimates of disease occurrence are essential for many of the other objectives. This basic information allows the costs of disease to be calculated, the relative importance of different diseases to be compared, comparison of the occurrence of disease by region, and changes in the occurrence over time to be observed. These estimates must therefore be made on a regular basis and be referable to spatially defined sub-populations. To be useful, estimates should be unbiased and of known precision.

The third task is to determine the epidemiology, geographical and temporal patterns, and risk factors associated with the major disease problems. Epidemiological studies to identify the natural history of the disease and quantify associations with risk factors are needed in order to formulate disease control strategies.

Finally it is necessary to assess the relative economic impact of the diseases present. Information on losses caused by disease or decreased production, combined with disease prevalence estimates can be used to calculate the economic impact of different diseases. This information is important for priority setting, and benefit-cost analysis of proposed disease control programs.

In addition to disease information basic ancillary (non-veterinary) information which may be used to provide a better basis for decision making may also be collected. A wide range of information can be used to support animal health decision making. Livestock population figures are essential for the calculation of rates (Martin *et al* 1987 p267). Other examples include data on livestock movement patterns, and veterinary infrastructure.

To help assess priorities and develop policies. Once basic animal health information has been collected, it must be used to set priorities for the use of resources for research or disease control programs. Priority setting is one of the major roles of veterinary services decision makers. The information provided by the animal health information system should be appropriate to enable decision makers to decide, for instance, which diseases or problems are significant enough to warrant the implementation of control programs. To assist with these decisions, the reports must present the information in a readily understandable manner. Clear priorities and sound information can aid more rational and informed national policy formulation and evaluation including not only policy on disease control programs, but also issues such as veterinary regulations and international trade.

To support the implementation of disease control programs. The system should also be able to provide continuous monitoring of carefully selected diseases, to assist in the development and evaluation of control programs. Monitoring implies the measuring of changes over time, which requires repeated measurements of key indicators. This information can be used to develop control programs for specific diseases, or to continuously evaluate the performance of existing control programs.

The system should be able to identify and respond to emerging diseases. Both exotic disease incursions and newly emerging diseases need to be identified quickly if effective action to limit their effects is to be taken.

To meet international reporting obligations. Finally, the information system must provide information necessary to meet international disease reporting requirements and to justify disease status claims for the purposes of international trade. The system of international trade in animals and animal products depends on the availability of reliable information regarding the disease status of trading partners. The Office Internationale des Epizooties (OIE) was set up to coordinate the international exchange of disease information. OIE member countries have a responsibility to provide reliable information on the presence or absence of significant livestock diseases. The creation of the World Trade Organisation, and the Agreement on the Application of Sanitary and Phytosanitary Measures (OIE and WHO, 1994) means that trading partners must be in a position to substantiate disease status claims using sound epidemiological information.

A range of different data is required to meet the needs of these four objectives, however all the data have one common feature – they all refer to an identifiable geographic location. Underlying each of these objectives is the need to take the spatial component of disease distribution into account.

Within this basic framework, there is a wide range of approaches involving varying levels of complexity that may be used to achieve these objectives. At the most complex level, this may involve the use of the system for research purposes, using advanced analyses, modelling and simulation to answer particular questions (for example, control program formulation). Before an animal health information system can be used effectively for this type of sophisticated research, it must first be able to meet the objectives in a more straightforward way, through the collection, management and reporting of the basic information required by the various users.

2.2.2 Components of an animal health information system

An optimal animal health information system should contain the following components (Martin *et al* 1987 p259).

Data gathering. Thrusfield (1995 p143-149) discusses a range of sources of veterinary data for an animal health information system. Those suitable for an animal health information system include notifiable disease reporting, routine diagnostic data, slaughterhouse records, sentinel herd monitoring systems, livestock population censuses, sentinel practice systems, disease control programme implementation and monitoring records and special surveys (Martin *et al* 1987 p259ff; Morris, 1976; Beal, 1983; Meier and Hauser 1996, Stark 1996,). As government veterinary services are reduced, there is likely to be an increasing reliance on information held by the private sector. A challenge will be to gain access to this information which is often regarded as commercially sensitive and therefore not available for general distribution.

Data collation. The collation of the collected data involves a series of administrative procedures to get the data from the animal or livestock owner to the place where it will be used. Most systems are based on the use of forms to record the data, and to transmit them to regional or national centres for collation.

Data storage and manipulation. Effective national animal health information systems must be able to handle a large amount of information efficiently. Paper-based systems exist, but are inefficient, and are severely limited in the volume of information they can handle and the uses to which the information can be put. Computerised systems, using a database management system are more common, even in developing countries. In order to store and manipulate spatially referenced data, geographical information systems, are required.

Data analysis. Appropriate analysis is required to convert data to information which can be used to assist animal health decision making. Data analysis is usually performed by computer, and can range from the simple calculation of totals and rates, to the determination of complicated statistical associations and the use of epidemiological models to predict the outcome of interventions.

Reporting. Once the results have been analysed they must be made available to those who need it. The information has value at many different levels – potential users include livestock owners, owner groups, cooperatives, or enterprise industry bodies, private veterinary services, agricultural product manufacturers, local, provincial and national government veterinary authorities, legislators, university and research organisations, trading partners, and international organisations (Martinez *et al*, 1992). A range of reporting approaches are usually required to pass on information to the many different users. For instance, government extension services may be used to communicate at the livestock owner level, annual reports and seminars at the government level, and standardised periodic report forms for international organisations. These five components are linked by a series of administrative procedures. As an example, the figure 2 below shows a schematic diagram of the data inputs for an animal health information system incorporating a geographical information system:

Figure 2

Data Inputs for an animal health information system

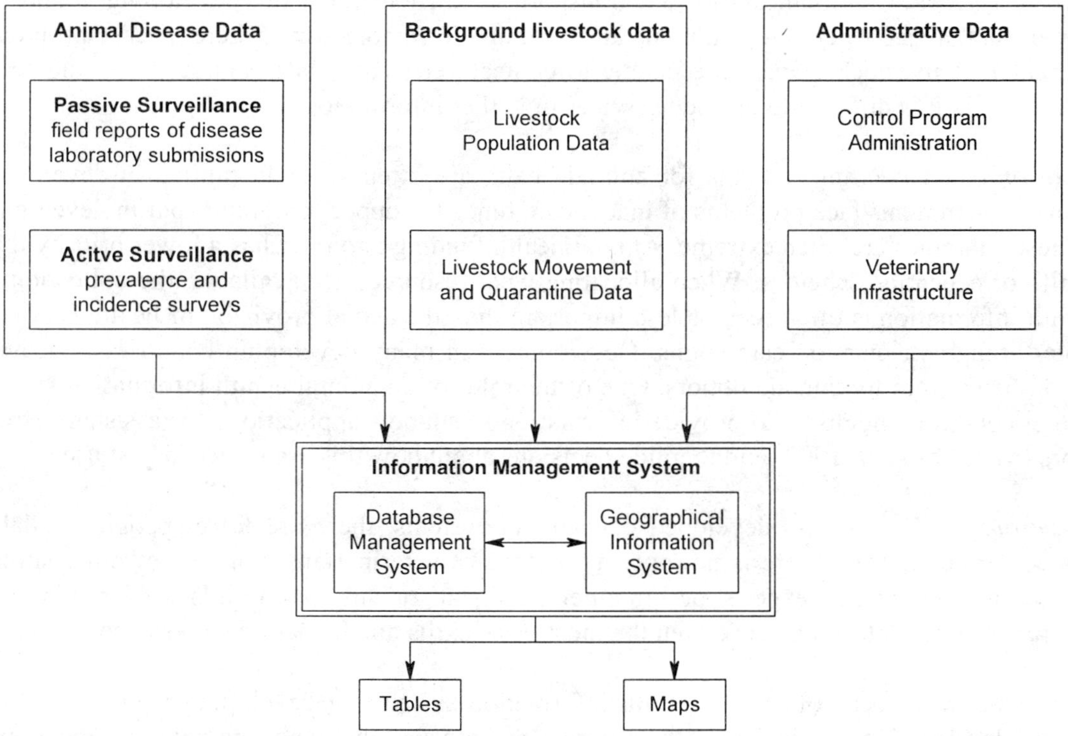

2.2.3 Animal health information systems in developing countries

The animal health information systems of developing countries serve a slightly different role and face vastly different challenges to those of developed countries. Despite these differences, the principles and philosophical approach remain the same.

Disease situation. The main disease problems faced by developed countries are increasingly either chronic diseases or production limiting diseases (Blood and Brightling, 1988). In developing countries, the main disease problems are often epidemic diseases that cause high morbidity and/or high mortality. While developed countries may never have experienced such diseases, or have eradicated them, many developing countries suffer high losses from epidemic diseases, and due to poor quarantine and uncontrolled livestock movement, new diseases continue to spread.

Dependence on agriculture. The economy of developing countries is often much more dependent on the agricultural sector, and livestock usually make an important contribution to this. For instance, in 1996, the proportion of USA's gross domestic product (GDP) made up by agriculture was 2% (CIA, 1997) whereas in Lao PDR it was 50%. In Lao PDR, 80% of the population are employed in agriculture as compared to 2.8% in the USA. The Lao government estimates that 22% of GDP comes from the livestock sector alone (Mekhagnomdara, 1996). The greater dependence on livestock means that livestock diseases of any sort have a much greater impact on the country as a whole.

Veterinary infrastructure. The veterinary infrastructure in many developing countries is often scant (Blood and Brightling, 1988). Veterinary services in developing countries are generally provided by government as there are very few private veterinary practices. The governments do not have the financial resources to employ sufficient skilled staff, nor do they have the resources to train their staff to a high level. As a result, most trained veterinarians working in government veterinary services work at policy or administrative levels. Field services are provided by para-veterinary staff with limited technical training or by village volunteers with virtually no training.

Physical infrastructure. Communications and transport are difficult in many developing countries, particularly in rural areas, where most animals are kept, and in remote areas where disease problems are often greater. If livestock owners are unable to contact veterinary staff, and staff are unable to access the livestock, it is difficult to provide services or gather information.

Financial resources. Government funds for animal health are often severely limited in developing countries. All governments face problems of inadequate funds to support programs, but in developing countries these shortages are often extreme. Animal health funding naturally has a lower priority than human health or education schemes. When allocating what resources are available, the collection of animal health information is often seen as less important than the actual provision of health services, for example through vaccination campaigns. Development in many developing countries is heavily dependent on funds from foreign aid donors. One of the roles of an animal health information system in developing countries should be to provide information to support applications for assistance from these donors (Martinez *et al*, 1992) and to guide decisions about how this assistance is best used.

Personnel resources. Due to less developed educational systems, there are fewer people available with the necessary expertise. There is not only a shortage of veterinarians, but also of other skilled staff such as computer systems experts, programmers, and statisticians. Due to a lack of training and infrastructure, veterinary staff may lack even the most basic skills due to lack of experience.

Information focus. The focus of animal health information systems in developing countries differs from that in developed countries, due to differences between the environments. In developed countries, the diseases of interest are mainly production diseases, and surveillance activities focus on detecting the introduction of exotic diseases or the substantiation of freedom from disease for international trade. Eradication programs are targeted at chronic diseases and diseases of public health significance. In developing countries the focus of the system is more on gathering information on what diseases are present, and the control or eradication of major epidemic diseases.

Integration of technology. As a result of limited financial and personnel resources, many developing countries have been unable to keep pace with changes in information technology. While complex computer-based information systems, including geographical information systems are commonplace in the developed world, many developing countries continue to use paper-based information systems.

New technologies require new skills, and pose new problems, such as the need for different types of data.

2.2.4 Examples of animal health information systems

Readily available published information on the structure and function of animal health information systems in developing countries is rather scarce, partly due to the lack of resources for development and research in this area. Another difficulty is that an animal health information system is hard to grasp and define, as it comprises a wide range of different components such as staff, forms, administrative procedures, information flows, hardware, software, analytical procedures, reports and publications. The following information has therefore been gathered from published and unpublished documents, and discussions with government veterinary staff.

Animal health information systems often evolve alongside the administrative information systems of the responsible organisations. Every organisation requires some form of structured information flow to organise and control its own activities. Administrative and animal health information systems are therefore often intertwined. This discussion deals only with the animal health component, but in reality, this division is not clear.

2.2.4.1 Asia-Pacific

Thailand. Thailand's animal health information system operates through an administrative hierarchy for the collection and transfer of data (Meephuch, in press). The Department of Livestock Development (DLD) in the Ministry of Agriculture is responsible for veterinary services. There is no single centralised division responsible for handling all animal health information. This task is shared primarily by the Disease Control Division, and the National Institute of Animal Health, although some information is collated, analysed and reported only at the regional level. Field services are coordinated through 9 regional offices, 76 provincial offices, and about 800 district offices. Most of the 60 000 villages have a volunteer (*asasamak*, or keyman). The volunteer is given basic animal health training, and is responsible for liaising with government staff and providing basic services for village livestock, such as vaccination. Animal health information handled by the DLD falls into six categories: diagnostic laboratory submissions, livestock populations, FMD and rabies outbreak reports, vaccine distribution, livestock movements, FMD surveillance activities and the agricultural census.

Lao PDR. Animal health in Lao PDR is the responsibility of the Animal Health Division in the Department of Livestock and Fisheries. Field veterinary services are organised through 18 provincial livestock offices, and 130 district offices. As in Thailand, there is a network of village volunteers (Village Veterinary Workers or VVWs) who take responsibility for animal health at the village level. This network is still under development, with about 6000 trained villagers in the country's 12 000 villages, of which only about 4000 are actively working. The animal health information system in Lao PDR is still in a very rudimentary stage (Vongthilath, in press). All records are paper based. Due to severe financial and infrastructure constraints, communication with the provinces is limited, and there is scant animal health information flow from many parts of the country. Information handled comprises diagnostic laboratory submissions, field disease reports, village livestock populations, livestock movements and vaccine distribution. Recently, a pilot system to handle all the routine reporting needs of the Animal Health Division has been developed (Sergeant *et al* 1997). This has involved development of modified reporting systems and establishment of a low cost national database with automated mapping facilities.

Indonesia. Indonesia's National Diseases Surveillance System is based primarily on the treatment records of semi-skilled village-based paraveterinarians, and on diagnostic test results. Problems with information management systems and the use of passively acquired data have lead to under-reporting, and data biases (Oka *et al*, 1992). Efforts are being made to incorporate data gathered through field investigations of livestock disease and productivity problems, based on simple standardised measures and sound epidemiological techniques (Hutabarat and Morris, 1997).

Cambodia. Cambodia's information system is similar in its level of development to that of Lao PDR (Chrea and Chhoeung, in press). There is a single central diagnostic laboratory. The epidemiology section has the responsibility of carrying out disease outbreak investigations and collecting specimens. Small-scale serosurveillance exercises have been undertaken in conjunction with aid projects (Forman and Leslie, 1997), but have not used statistically sound techniques. Standard laboratory submission forms exist, but infrastructure, communications and security problems severely limit the number of specimens and outbreak reports received. There are currently no internal livestock movement checkpoints nor any international quarantine checkpoints.

Vietnam. Vietnam's information system benefits from the more strongly developed veterinary infrastructure than that of its neighbours in Cambodia or Lao PDR (Lai Thi Kim and Thai Thi Thuy, in press). Vietnam has a three tiered laboratory system, with provincial, regional and national diagnostic laboratories. An array of standardised report forms are used for laboratory submissions and field reports. Village livestock population data is collected twice yearly by the Ministry of Investment and Planning. Livestock movement checkpoints record international (20 checkpoints) and internal (45 checkpoints) movements. Disease eradication programs are currently underway for anthrax, FMD and rabies, but these are not supported by any active surveillance programme. The field infrastructure is made up of field veterinarians, veterinary technicians and vaccinators. A Sector of Animal Health Information Management has recently been established. Despite the extensive infrastructure and the large amount of information collected at various levels, collation, analysis and reporting of this information is still at an early stage of development. The system is almost completely paper-based.

The Philippines. The Philippines has a relatively developed veterinary infrastructure and animal health information system (Abila and Joco, in press). Disease information is based primarily on laboratory submissions and field reports from disease outbreak investigations. Serosurveillance is used from time to time for target diseases, but surveys may lack statistical validity. Information is managed by the Disease Intelligence Section of the Animal Health Division and the Epidemiology Section of the Philippines Animal Health Centre. Veterinary services are primarily under the control of provincial governors, leading to difficulties in the coordination of national disease control programs. Key data are maintained on computer spreadsheets, and a village-based health and production data collection system is being trialed (Abila, 1997). Recently, a comprehensive information system to support the national FMD eradication program has been developed. This system handles all information relevant to FMD control including demographics, personnel, FMD surveillance activities, quarantine check point activities and vaccine distribution and use. The system produces both tabular and map based reports of a variety of types.

Malaysia. Malaysia is one of the most developed countries in the South East Asian region. The country's information system is relatively advanced, with computerised management of diagnostic laboratory and field veterinary services records (Kadir *et al*, 1997). This information is linked to a computerised mapping system for the automated generation of disease maps (but not a fully functional GIS). Unlike in the other countries in the region, private veterinarians play a significant role in delivery of services. This causes some problems in the quality of information available to the information system. Serosurveillance is used at times for target diseases.

Australia. Reporting of information on Australia's animal health status is effected through the National Animal Health Information System (NAHIS) which is jointly funded by government and animal industries. The purpose of the NAHIS is to provide timely and accurate summary information on Australia's animal health status as well as animal disease surveillance and control activities and capabilities. Data for the NAHIS comes from a variety of sources including government and non-government agencies and is channelled through State/Territory and Commonwealth Coordinators whose roles are defined in a business plan. The main outputs include a small database for textual and summary numerical data on animal diseases; a web site to permit remote anonymous access to the information (www.brs.gov.au/aphb/aha); quarterly reports known as "Animal Health Surveillance Quarterly"; an annual report known as "Animal Health in Australia"; routine reports to the Office International des Epizooties, Food and Agriculture Organisation of the United Nations and the World Health Organisation; and ad hoc reports as required (Baldock and Garner 1998).

2.2.4.2 Africa

Nigeria. Nigeria's information system, the National Disease Reporting System (NRDS) is based solely on passive disease reporting (Ogundipe *et al*, 1989). Information is collected via a three tiered hierarchy – local veterinarians, state monitoring offices, and a central National Disease Recording Centre. There is compulsory notification of 113 diseases. Disease reports or specimen submissions are made on one of ten forms for the purpose, and are accompanied by map references for the origin of the report.

Namibia. A computerised animal health information system has been developed in Namibia (Biggs and Hare, 1994; Hare and Biggs, 1996). This system uses incident-based (passive) reporting as well as routine farm visits to most of the farms in the country.

Senegal. Senegal has introduced a surveillance system for health and productivity of small ruminants, using individual animal identification and record keeping (Faugère *et al*, 1991). Non-random, selected herds are monitored with fortnightly visits.

Other African systems. Sollod and Stem (1991) describe the implementation of an animal health information system for transhumant livestock populations in Africa, based on the "Vetscouts", members of migratory communities who receive basic training and are responsible for disease reporting. Many countries in Africa are involved in active surveillance as part of their participation in the Pan African Rinderpest Campaign, for example Mali (Tounkara *et al*, 1990), Gambia (Touray, 1990) and Nigeria (Ezeokoli *et al*, 1990). While these activities are essential for that particular disease eradication programme, and are valuable in developing the experience of veterinary staff, they do not form an integral part of national animal health information systems.

2.2.5 Regional information systems

In addition to the various national systems described, there are a number of regional animal health information systems (handling information from a number of countries). These regional systems generally collate data from national-level veterinary services and report to other countries in the region, with the aim of preventing trans-boundary disease spread, and the coordination of disease control and eradication programs. Foremost amongst these systems is the OIE's global reporting system (Blajan, 1979; Blajan and Chillaud, 1991; King, 1994) for the distribution of reports about 15 high priority (List A) and about 90 lower priority (List B) diseases amongst 136 member countries.

The Carribean Animal and Plant Health Information Network (CARAPHIN) links 23 Carribean countries for sharing information on common animal and plant disease threats (Bernardo *et al*, 1991; Waltner-Toews *et al*, 1991).

In Southeast Asia, the Animal Health and Production Information System for ASEAN (AHPISA) is in the process of setting up a coordinated regional information system (Hutabarat *et al*, 1994; Bedard *et al*, 1997). Part of the role of the OIE sub-commission for FMD South-East Asia is to coordinate the exchange of information about this disease to support a regional control and eradication scheme (OIE, 1996).

The Pan American Foot and Mouth Disease Centre has established a regional information system for vesicular diseases (Olascoaga, 1982) throughout central and south America. This compiles data from national information systems using passive surveillance and regular weekly situation reports. Participating countries have well structured systems for the routine flow of information from the district to the central level (OIE, 1982a, b).

2.3 Active surveillance

Surveillance activities are an integral part of a national animal health information system. In the International Animal Health Code of the OIE, disease surveillance is defined as: *the continuous investigation of a given population to detect the occurrence of disease for control purposes, which may involve testing of a part of the population.*

A variety of names have been used to describe different types of surveillance activities. Terms such as *passive surveillance* and *active surveillance* are commonly used, but it is not always clear what they mean. Briefly, *passive surveillance* is the **secondary use** of routinely collected data which was generated for some other purpose while *active surveillance* is the routine collection of data whose **primary purpose** is for surveillance. Thus, use of laboratory diagnostic records would be seen as *passive surveillance* while results from a survey to reliably estimate the prevalence of a particular disease is an example of *active surveillance.* In reality, there are many ways that different surveillance activities can be described.

In contrast to passive surveillance, active surveillance involves the active collection of accurate and representative field data on the health of the livestock population (Martin *et al* 1987 p 261). Active surveillance data incorporated into an animal health information system is collected in order to meet the requirements of the users of the system. In order to maximise the value of active surveillance it must be based on statistically sound survey techniques (Hueston, 1993). As only a small sample of the total population is examined, the population at risk in the sample can be easily counted. Bias is avoided by the use of probability sampling techniques, and appropriate analysis provides valid measures of the precision of estimates.

In its broadest sense, active surveillance encompasses any form of active data collection for surveillance. In human epidemiology, the term is sometimes applied to active case-seeking, through the use of multiple data sources, and a similar meaning has been applied in veterinary epidemiology (Anderson, 1982). Surveillance systems based on the compilation of results from many herd-level monitoring systems have been developed. One example from Canada is the Animal Productivity and Health Information Network (APHIN) (Thrusfield, 1995 p163). This system combines data from participating individual pig, beef and dairy computerised herd health and productivity schemes, and combines them with other data sources such as abattoir and diagnostic laboratory results. As a non-random sample of herds are involved in the scheme, results cannot be extrapolated to the wider population. In the present thesis, the term active surveillance is limited to the use of population-based survey techniques to collect data which enables the calculation of valid estimates of disease occurrence.

Last (1988 p125) defines surveillance as "ongoing scrutiny, generally using methods distinguished by their practicability, uniformity, and frequently their rapidity, rather than by their accuracy. Its main purpose is to detect changes in trend or distribution in order to initiate investigative or control measures." For developing countries there is a pressing need to use practical, rapid techniques rather than extremely precise techniques.

2.3.1 Survey sampling

As statistical sampling techniques are a central part of active surveillance, some background to, and justification of the importance of, survey sampling is warranted.

There are two main types of surveys. A census is a survey in which every member of the population is examined (Kish, 1995 p18). Censuses are rarely used to gather animal disease information on a large scale, as they are prohibitively expensive. Censuses have the advantage that inference from the results is not necessary, and that the results, at least in theory, have no statistical uncertainty associated with them.

Sample surveys differ from censuses in that only a proportion of animals in the population (a sample) is examined (Levy and Lemeshow, 1991 p2). This means that the survey may be much simpler and cheaper to perform. The drawback with sample surveys is that they do not provide an exact measure of the level of disease. The value of sample surveys is that they allow one to estimate the prevalence (or other value of interest) in the population, using inference. The validity of this inference depends on how representative the sample is of the study population.

The accuracy of an estimation technique (a way of taking a sample, and calculating the estimate from that sample) is described in terms of two measures: bias and precision (Thrusfield, 1995 p134). Bias is the difference between the expected value produced by the estimation technique and the true value in the population. One common cause of bias is the way in which the sample is chosen, sampling bias. Precision, measured by variance, indicates the theoretical spread of the different results that would be obtained by repeated surveys of the same population. The main factor which affects the precision of an estimate is the sample size.

2.3.2 Sampling methods

There are many ways to select a sample from a population for a survey. The desirable characteristics of a sample are that it:

- is representative of the study population, to allow inference back to that population;
- produces unbiased estimates;
- produces estimates of known precision.

A representative sample is a sample that has the same characteristics as the study population, with regard to the value of interest. A method is therefore needed to select a sample of animals, so that they are very likely to have the same characteristics as the study population.

Two different groups of sampling techniques exist: non-probability and probability. Probability sampling techniques are those in which each member of the population has a known, non-zero probability of being selected in the sample (Kish, 1995 p20). Non-probability sampling is a technique in which this is not the case (Martin *et al*, 1987 p25) . These two groups are considered below.

Non-probability sampling techniques include convenience samples, purposive samples, and haphazard samples. Convenience samples are chosen because they are easy, quick or inexpensive to collect. Purposive or judgmental sampling involves the selection of "typical" animals in an effort to achieve a representative or balanced sample. Haphazard samples are chosen with no fixed purpose or reason, in an attempt to imitate random sampling. All non-probability sampling techniques carry a great risk of producing biased estimates. It is not possible to estimate variance using a non-probability sampling technique.

Probability sampling is based on the concept of randomness, and the use of random numbers (Martin *et al* 1987 p25). Random numbers are sets of numbers in a certain range such that each number in the range has the same probability of appearing in the set. Simple random sampling is the most basic form of probability sampling. Each member of the population has the same probability of being selected.

Systematic sampling is often more practical than simple random sampling. Using systematic sampling, prior identification of the animals is not necessary. Animals are selected using a fixed sampling interval, calculated as the population size divided by the desired sample size.

Stratified sampling involves dividing the population up into separate, exclusive strata, and sampling from each. There are two main reasons for using stratification. Firstly, it enables us to calculate estimates not only for the whole population, but for each stratum as well. The second reason for using stratification is that it may produce more precise results (by creating low within-stratum variability, and high between-stratum variability).

The last forms of random sampling to be considered, multi-stage and cluster sampling, are the most complex. In simple random sampling, all animals need to be first identified. In systematic sampling, they need to be "lined up" in some sort of sequence for sampling. For large-scale livestock surveys, multi-stage sampling is usually necessary (Cochran, 1977 p233).

Multi-stage sampling gathers the animals into convenient groups (Levy and Lemeshow, 1991 p175-182). For instance, in two-stage sampling, groups of animals (e.g. villages) are randomly selected and then individual animals are randomly chosen from the selected groups. When all animals in a group are examined in the final stage, this technique is called cluster sampling. Multi-stage and cluster samples have two distinct advantages: they are easier to plan, as a complete list of all animals is not needed, only primary sampling units; and they are more practical for the field work team, as fewer sites need to be visited. The disadvantages are that the results may not be as precise as with simple random sampling, and the formulae for analysis of the data can be very complex. Sampling strategies in which each animal in the population has the same probability of selection, known as self-weighting samples, are generally the easiest to analyse (Levy and Lemeshow, 1991 p126).

A wide variety of other designs have been applied to the problem of large area surveys, for example the use of three or more stages of sampling, multiple levels of stratification (e.g. (Kish, 1995 p359ff), or abattoir sampling. Each different sampling strategy is a compromise between many competing factors, for instance data accuracy, cost, ease of field operations, and complexity of analytical procedures. Increasing the levels of stratification generally places a greater demand on the amount and quality of information required about the population before the survey can be designed. Increasing the number of stages makes field operations simpler, but may decrease the statistical efficiency of the survey, and certainly increases the complexity of analytical formulae. In practice, statisticians faced with the analysis of survey designs including more than two stages, generally abandon traditional sampling theory, and use bootstrapping or related techniques to calculate variance estimates (Levy and Lemeshow, 1991 p280). This approach allows extremely complicated survey designs to be applied, but requires a reasonable level of understanding of statistical theory and the use of powerful computer hardware and software. These considerations mean that the use of more complex sampling designs are beyond the capacity of the veterinary services of most developing countries, without the assistance of external statistical expertise for survey design and analysis.

Abattoir surveys have been used to assess the health status of large populations (Robertson and Blackmore, 1985; Scott-Orr, 1985; Ramsay *et al*, 1995a). Abattoir surveys have the advantages that large numbers of animals from a wide area are collected together in one place, and collection of blood and other specimens is relatively quick and simple. The disadvantages of these surveys are that abattoir surveys represent a form of convenience sampling: the reference population is usually unable to be clearly defined, and animals sent to abattoirs are not representative of the total population. These problems make it impossible to calculate unbiased estimates of disease prevalence. In some circumstances, the convenience of the use of abattoir surveys may outweigh the limitations of the data that can be collected.

2.3.3 Sampling to detect disease or substantiate disease freedom

The prevention of disease spread through the movement of live animals can be reduced by diagnostic testing and certification by appropriate authorities. For terrestrial animals such as cattle, serological tests are available for many diseases and every animal in a shipment may be tested. However, such a strategy may be impractical in some instances and only a sample of animals may be tested to decide if the group is infected or not with a certain level of confidence.

What is not commonly realised is that testing for disease at the group level incorporates a number of factors additional to those relevant to testing at the individual animal level. Thus, techniques such as serology which may be highly sensitive and specific at the individual animal level can still result in misclassification of a high proportion of groups where only a small proportion are tested.

At the individual animal level, diagnostic test performance is determined by its sensitivity and specificity. From an epidemiological perspective, sensitivity is the proportion of animals infected with the agent of interest who test positive while specificity is the proportion of uninfected animals who test negative. Additional factors which come into play when a group of animals is to be classified are the number of animals tested, the prevalence of disease in the group and the level of statistical confidence required that the group is truly negative. The only way to be 100% confident that no animals comprising a particular group are infected with a particular agent is to test every animal in the group with a diagnostic test which has perfect sensitivity and specificity. However, if only a low proportion of individual animals in the group are infected and only a small number are tested there can be quite a high chance that infected groups will be misclassified as uninfected. The table below shows the number of infected animals which can be in a group of 100,000 despite a sample testing negative using a test with perfect sensitivity and specificity at the individual animal level (Cannon and Roe 1982).

	No. of infected animals which could be in the group despite the sample testing negative (two levels of confidence shown)	
No. of animals in sample tested from group of 100,000 and found negative	**95%**	**99%**
100	2,950	4,499
500	596	915
1,000	298	458
10,000	29	44

The situation is further complicated where the diagnostic test being used has imperfect sensitivity and specificity and where two stage sampling is used to select animals for testing (eg a number of farms or villages are initially selected and then a number of animals chosen from each selected farm or village) which is the case for many of those in use in livestock. Methods to choose the appropriate numbers to sample in these circumstances have been developed (Jordan 1995, Cameron and Baldock 1998a,b)

2.3.4 Sentinel herd systems

Regular monitoring of sentinel herds is a form of active surveillance suited to those diseases where incidence data is required and where the disease is fairly common. Sentinel herds are not suitable for sporadic diseases. They have commonly been used for arbovirus monitoring in cattle and the basic technique has been described by St George (1980). In summary, uninfected healthy young cohorts of animals are periodically examined and bled for serology until there is a change in their status. Observations may also be made on possible explanatory factors such as weather, vegetation and the occurrence of vectors.

Data from such systems has been used for a variety of purposes such as incidence of seroconversion to bluetongue virus in cattle (Shaw 1992; Ward *et al* 1995), incidence of bovine ephemeral fever (St George 1985) incidence of trypansomiasis in cattle (Paling *et al* 1987) and association of Rift Valley fever infections with vegetation changes (Davies *et al* 1992).

2.3.5 Sentinel practice systems

This is another form of active surveillance. Though commonly used in the surveillance of common human diseases, sentinel veterinary practice systems have a poor record of performance. The problem appears mainly to lie in failure of veterinary practices to provide comprehensive reports over a sustained period of time. However, some systems do work. In Switzerland, information on a number of important equine diseases is obtained through a practice network (Meier and Hauser 1996). In Australia, a pilot system is being evaluated in the State of Victoria for a small range of equine conditions (Dr P Ellis, personal communication).

2.3.6 Remote sensing

Data of various types gathered either by satellite or aerial photography can be used to provide information relevant to animal diseases. Analysing and interpreting such data is usually computer intensive and in some cases may be quite expensive. Nevertheless, in some circumstances, use of such data may be a cost-effective means of disease surveillance. Remotely sensed data has been used for a range of purposes from identification of villages for surveys through to complex disease predictions. Cameron (1997) used satellite and aerial photographs combined with a GIS as a survey tool for a single province in Lao PDR. At the other end of the spectrum, Estrada-Pena (1999) used data satellite data together with geostatistics (cokriging) to model the correlation between the temperature and vegetation variables and the distribution of the cattle tick, *Boophilus microplus* at a continental level.

The main applications have been in using data such as plant cover, surface temperature, moisture indices and brightness in the analysis of the distribution of vector-borne diseases (Washino and Wood 1994, Kitron 1998). Such techniques have recently been applied to ectoparasites (Dale *et al* 1998, Flasse *et al* 1998), malaria (Sharma and Srivastava 1997, Hay *et al* 1998), filariasis (Hassan *et al* 1998), Rift Valley fever (Linthicum *et al* 1990) and Lyme disease (Dister *et al* 1997

2.3.7 Active surveillance in developed countries

Survey techniques based on probability sampling have been in common use for many decades. However they have been used mainly in research and one-off surveys, and have been seen as relatively time consuming and expensive. The OIE has advocated the use of active surveillance to complement passive data collection systems such as laboratory databases and disease notifications (Blajan, 1979). If such techniques are to be incorporated into a disease surveillance system, surveys need to be conducted on a regular basis (depending on the information requirements), and be able to provide results rapidly. Animal health administrators in many developed countries have realised that the passive surveillance systems based on laboratory submissions and disease notifications are inadequate for providing valid measures of disease incidence. The most completely documented use of active surveillance for animal health comes from the United States of America (Alderink, 1985; Dahl, 1985; Hoffsis, 1985; King, 1985, 1988; Mulhern, 1985; Farrar, 1988). Attempts have been made to introduce a range of surveillance systems in the USA over the last 50 years, initially based on passive reporting systems (McCallon and Beal, 1982b; Glosser, 1988). The needs for statistically sound data (Poppensiek, 1985; King, 1986) on prevalence or incidence, trends and economic impacts of disease meant that data collection using probability sampling was required (Beal, 1983; Diesch, 1988). The National Animal Health Monitoring Scheme (NAHMS) uses active surveillance in the form of a series of large surveys to provide it with animal health and production information. The unit of interest is the farm, and a two-stage stratified sampling strategy is used, selecting county with probability proportional to size at the first stage, and farm using simple random sampling at the second (Martin 1983; Kelch and New, 1993; Losinger *et al* 1998). The NAHMS represents one of the most comprehensive national-level animal health information systems to routinely incorporate active surveillance. Unfortunately, the use of statistically sound sampling techniques is not enough to ensure an effective system. No formal cost-benefit analysis of the NAHMS has been published, and it is possible that the costs outweigh the value of the data. In many other countries, the implementation of structured active surveillance programs is at a less advanced stage.

In Australia, animal health information has long been based on passive data sources (Rolfe, 1985; Andrews, 1988), although the need for active surveillance is becoming apparent (Morris, 1976; Garner and Nunn, 1991). The brucellosis and tuberculosis eradication campaign (BTEC) endeavoured to maintain complete data on the status of every herd in the country (Cannon, 1993). This could perhaps be considered as a form of active surveillance, however repeated testing of every animal in the country is prohibitively expensive in most situations. Active surveillance in the form of regular national serological surveys to provide high-quality data on selected diseases, and the use of sera to establish a representative serum bank has been advocated (Garner, 1993). The current Australian national animal health information system relies on the compilation of data gathered by the veterinary authorities in each state. Disease information is primarily incidence-based and acquired through passive reporting (Garner, 1997). Some states are introducing active surveillance systems to complement their passive data sources. For example, in Queensland, a pilot programme using structured active surveillance in the extensive beef industry has been successfully completed (Baldock, 1995; Queensland Department of Primary Industries, 1995; Black *et al*, 1997). This programme uses both farm visits for specimen collection and farmer-recorded observations from a random sample of beef farms to collect representative data on 22 priority diseases.

The Canadian national animal health information system is similarly based on the use of passively acquired data, as well as serosurveillance collecting data using convenience sampling. Active surveillance using valid sampling techniques is being used to monitor the health and productivity of swine herds (Morley, 1988).

In Switzerland, a pilot project to develop health and productivity profiles for dairy cows was established (Stärk, 1996). A stratified random sample was chosen, specimens collected and health events recorded by farmers over a 15 month period. The representativeness of this sample may be questioned, as only 42% of farms contacted agreed to participate, potentially introducing a selection bias. However, comparison of baseline parameters from participating and non-participating herds showed little difference (Stärk *et al*, 1994). Statistically based sample surveys have also been used to substantiate freedom from infectious bovine rhinotracheitis (IBR) and enzootic bovine leucosis (EBL).

In New Zealand, passive data collection forms the basis for most animal health information (McKenzie and Thompson, 1991). There is the provision for the implementation of specific epidemiological studies to gather valid disease occurrence estimates if this information is required. However, published examples of such surveys indicate that non-random sampling is sometimes used, and the results may therefore be biased (Thornton and Motha, 1995).

Great Britain's animal health information system is heavily dependent on passively acquired data, but uses a system of herd testing for the eradication of brucellosis and tuberculosis similar to that used in Australia (Scudamore, 1988).

Animal health information in most developed countries is still largely based on passive data collection. The few systems incorporating routine active surveillance based on statistically sound sampling techniques have demonstrated that it is possible to use this approach to gather reliable animal health data.

Chapter 3.2.13 (Bovine Spongiform Encephalopathy) of the OIE International Animal Health Code specifically describes how active surveillance is to be undertaken for the continuous demonstration of freedom from BSE for free countries. Countries such as Argentina, Canada, USA, Australia and New Zealand which export large quantities of beef, now have in place active surveillance programs for BSE based on the OIE Code. In Australia, at least, essential data from BSE surveillance are held in a national database which can be queried over the internet.

2.3.8 Active surveillance in developing countries

The active surveillance techniques implemented in the animal health information systems of several developed countries are certainly able to provide the type of reliable data required. However the systems are relatively expensive to run, and require a great deal of expertise to manage. In developing countries, these costs may be prohibitive. Similarly the time, man-power and expertise required for such surveys may not be available.

Work in the fields of human health and development in developing countries offers suggestions of how these surveillance systems may be adapted to suit local conditions. The Expanded Programme for Immunisation (EPI) run by the World Health Organisation faced the problem of assessing vaccination coverage rates in developing countries, and developed a range of techniques for Rapid Epidemiological Assessment (REA) (Smith, G.S., 1989). These techniques include inexpensive, rapid survey techniques using a two-stage cluster sampling strategy. REA cluster surveys use a relatively small sample size (210) distributed amongst 30 sites (selected with probability proportional to size) with 7 people in each (the "30 by 7" design). Although the data produced from such a small survey is not very precise (aiming at a confidence interval of ± 10%) it is unbiased, of known precision and can be quickly collected (Anker, 1991). The advantages of this design for developing countries are that it is operationally simple, inexpensive and reasonably robust (Henderson and Sundaresan, 1982). Considerable research has gone into evaluating this design, and there have been a number of suggestions for modifications or improvements (Lemeshow and Robinson, 1985; Bennett *et al*, 1991; Harris and Lemeshow, 1991; Turner *et al*, 1996). One area that has gained some attention is the use of portable computers for rapid data collection and analysis (Bertrand, 1985; Birkett, 1988; Frerichs, 1989; Frerichs and Tar Tar, 1989).

Another rich source of techniques for use in developing countries comes from the field of Participatory Rural Appraisal (PRA) (Chambers *et al*, 1989; Mikkelsen, 1995). While more often applied to general community development projects, some of the data collection techniques used may well be applied to active surveillance for animal health.

There are few published examples of the use of active surveillance for animal health in developing countries. In Mexico, active surveillance has been used to collect randomized samples for targeted livestock diseases (Levaro and Guillen, 1983), although details of sampling techniques are not given. The Pan African Rinderpest Campaign (PARC) established recommendations for serosurveillance, based on statistically valid sample surveys (Tyler, 1990). The use of these methods has been reported in various countries, including Gambia (Touray, 1990), Mali (Tounkara *et al*, 1990) , Ethiopia (IAEA, 1992) and Nigeria (Ezeokoli *et al*, 1990). Internationally recognised standards for rinderpest surveillance now exist and are regularly updated (OIE 1998). These standards outline the criteria required to show that a zone or country is free from rinderpest as well as the process required for the declaration of freedom from rinderpest with more detail available in the *Recommended Procedures for Disease and Serological Surveillance as part of the Global Rinderpest Eradication Programme - GREP* (FAO/IAEA 1993). A similar international standard exists for contagious bovine pleuropneumonia (OIE 1997a). These are discussed further below.

In Thailand and the Philippines active surveillance using serology to monitor the effectiveness of mass vaccination is now a routine component of the FMD campaigns in those countries. Clearly, there may be other developing countries in the process of adopting active surveillance, which have not been reported in the literature. However, personal communications with national veterinary staff indicate that in at least, Myanmar, Lao PDR, Cambodia and Vietnam there is no statistically sound routine programme of active surveillance to collect data for incorporation into the national animal health information systems of these countries. Each country has been involved in surveillance for FMD, but these surveys either have been one-off efforts as part of bilaterally funded projects, or have no statistically sound basis to their design (resulting in biased estimates), or both.

There are a number of possible reasons for this failure of developing countries to adopt active surveillance as part of their national animal health information systems:

- lack of skills base. The veterinary staff may not have the epidemiological training required to realise the need for active surveillance. They many not appreciate the value of data for disease control purposes.
- lack of resources. The veterinary services may not have sufficient funds to implement active surveillance programs.
- lack of training and information. The veterinary staff may not have had access to sources of information on how to implement effective active surveillance.
- lack of statistical expertise. The complexity of sampling designs and analysis formulae may be an obstacle if veterinary staff do not have access to statistical expertise.
- lack of infrastructure. The veterinary infrastructure (provincial, district and village staff) or the physical infrastructure (e.g. roads) may be inadequate for field surveillance work.
- lack of motivation. Veterinary authorities may not believe in the relevance of active surveillance for developing countries, as there have been few examples of how it has been successfully implemented for the benefit of the country.

2.3.9 Active surveillance for rinderpest and CBPP

The OIE has developed international standards for surveillance for two diseases: Rinderpest (OIE 1998) and Contagious Bovine Pleuropneumonia (CBPP) (OIE 1997a).

The stated purpose of these standards is *"to provide evidence that a country or region is free from disease or infection"* and that *"disease surveillance should be implemented by both:*
a) a system of reporting any signs of disease activity which come to the notice of Veterinary Services or livestock owners; and

b) an active program of statistically selected samples from host populations in order to detect clinical signs or other indications of the occurrence of the disease or transmission of infection."

In demonstrating that a country or zone is free of disease it will be necessary to conduct a surveillance program that would have a very high probability of detecting the disease if it were present. According to the CBPP guidelines surveillance should include a combination of clinical, pathological, serological and microbiological methods based on an epidemiological approach. The mix of procedures will depend on the specific circumstances of the country or zone.

It is therefore clear that the surveillance system will need to include both passive and active elements. The herd is the sampling unit. A sampling unit for the purposes of disease investigation and surveillance is defined as a group of animals in sufficiently close contact that individuals in the group would be at approximately equal risk of coming in contact with the disease agent if there were an infectious animal in the group. Under the OIE standards, disease surveillance activities must be conducted on populations stratified according to the management system, and by herd size. Herds are to be selected by proper random statistical procedures for each stratum.

For both diseases, the guidelines on serological surveillance suggest that sample sizes must be sufficient to provide a 95% probability of detecting evidence of the disease if it were present in 1% of herds. As the number of samples required will be affected by the sensitivity of the test used, the sample size must be adjusted to allow for any lack of sensitivity in the testing procedure. Cattle and any other susceptible domestic species *must be included* in the sero-surveillance program. Wild susceptible species *must be sampled where possible* and domestic stock in contact with them *should be sampled intensively.*

While both of these documents provide excellent guidance on likely surveillance requirements, it is important to appreciate that they are both written from the perspective of a previously-infected country or zone wanting to be recognised as free following a control/eradication program.

Some countries which have been free of CBP for many years such as Switzerland still maintain active an active surveillance programme in the face of some risk of incursion from other European countries (Stark *et al* 1995).

2.4 Geographical information systems (GIS)

A GIS is a specialised computer database, which handles two types of information. Firstly it stores geographical information, the location of features, be they countries, administrative boundaries, rivers, roads, villages, or farms. Anything that has a physical location can be stored in a GIS. This first type of information is usually derived from maps, but may come from other sources, such as remote sensing (e.g. satellite images, aerial photography), or global positioning system (GPS) units. The second type of data stored in a GIS is called attribute data. This describes the attributes of the geographical features, or what they are like. Attributes can take any form, for example, the attributes of a village may include the name, the number of each species of animals present, diseases that have occurred, the average titre of the animals to a particular pathogen, feed available and so on. What makes a GIS different from a standard database is its ability to perform spatial analysis on the information stored. The spatial relationship between features and their associated attributes can be analysed to reveal underlying patterns. GIS technology can be applied to any situation in which data can be linked to a spatial location.

2.4.1 Role of GIS in animal health information systems

Data integration. Data integration involves the combination of data from two or more data sources, and the analysis of the combined data. For instance, data on village animal populations, village vaccine usage, and village disease outbreaks may be currently available, but in separate systems. If these three data sources were integrated, then population, vaccination and disease history could be analysed together. This would yield village level vaccine coverage rates (the number of animals vaccinated divided by the total number of animals). Vaccine coverage rates could then be related to disease history to assess vaccine effectiveness. On their own, the separate data sources are unable to provide this important information, but when integrated, the analysis is simple.

Any computerised relational database is able to achieve this type of data integration. In general it is achieved by linking two databases on the basis of a common key. In this example, the key may be a unique village identifier.

Efficiently linking geographical and attribute information is a central part of the function of a GIS. As a result, most GIS have very powerful, and simple to use data linking capabilities. This makes them well suited to the task of integrating the many different data sources that are required in an animal health information system.

Incorporating geographical data. One of the objectives of an animal health information system is to provide information that provides a better understanding of the epidemiology of disease. An important component of the epidemiology of a disease is the distribution of that disease in relation to a number of factors, such as species, age, sex, time and so on. One of the most important of these factors is the disease's distribution in relation to space, or its geographical distribution (Garner and Nunn, 1991). Traditional tools for epidemiological data management and analysis are very poorly equipped to handle information on the geographical distribution of disease, as the relationships between adjacent or distant areas cannot be examined. Traditional non-spatial database management systems can handle storage and analysis of the other factors. However, the use of a GIS offers the ability to include the spatial distribution of disease in the analysis of all the other factors.

While an understanding of the spatial distribution of disease is important for a full appreciation of the epidemiology of the disease, this information is even more important for some of the other roles of an animal health information system. To effectively support disease control and eradication programs, the spatial distribution of the disease and the susceptible population must be understood. Spatial patterns of livestock movement are able to help predict risk of disease spread. The establishment of a disease-free zone for international trade purposes requires a clear understanding of the spatial distribution of disease and risk factors in and around the zone.

Examination of the spatial component of animal health data yields another important benefit of GIS – the ability to quickly identify data errors. Missing and out-of-range data are easily identified when the data is mapped.

Currently, in many countries, spatial data are managed with the use of manually prepared disease maps. The level of detail and accuracy, time taken for preparation, and absence of analysis severely weaken the value of these manually prepared disease maps.

Improved reporting. Information on disease distribution is currently reported in the form of tables in monthly or annual reports, usually reporting number of cases per province or district. This information is difficult to interpret. Disease maps supplement this type of reporting. Maps are able to convey the relative levels of disease graphically, through the use of colour or different symbols. They also convey the relationships between different geographical areas. The message conveyed by a well prepared disease map is able to be understood in seconds, whereas the same data in tabular form may not be able to be properly understood at all. While a GIS is able to provide tabular summaries and charts, the main output is in the form of maps. The production of accurate attractive, well-presented disease maps can be completely automated, and achieved in seconds, given a database of up-to-date information.

The powerful analytical capabilities of a GIS enable more useful information to be presented in map form than just the number of cases of disease. When linked with population data, incidence rates, and relative risk maps can be produced, providing a much greater insight into the distribution of disease. Another key advantage of a GIS for improving reporting of animal health information is that maps can be used interactively. The user may zoom in to areas of particular interest, increase or decrease the amount if information presented simultaneously, query particular features to determine the actual value of attributes, or perform *ad hoc* analysis. A GIS is therefore well suited as a tool for providing animal health decision makers with the information they require.

2.4.2 Adoption of GIS

Many authors have recommended either the ability to manage spatial data, or the specific inclusion of a GIS in an animal health information system (Rolfe, 1985; Blood and Brightling, 1988; Morley, 1988; Sharma, 1994; Thrusfield, 1995 p54-57). GIS have been successfully applied to a number of specific problems in veterinary epidemiology, such as estimating the risk of East Coast fever to livestock in Africa (Lessard *et al*, 1988) and the analysis of chemical residue data from abattoirs (Van der Logt *et al*, 1994), to examine the epidemiology of tuberculosis in possums (Pfeiffer and Morris, 1994), or of Aujeszky's disease in pigs (Marsh *et al*, 1991a; Belfrage *et al*, 1994; McGinn *et al*, 1994). One of the more common uses of the technology has been as an aid in the control of disease outbreaks especially FMD (Sanson *et al*, 1991a, b, 1994).

There are however relatively few examples of the inclusion of a GIS as an integral part of an animal health information system. In South America, the Pan American Foot and Mouth Disease Centre uses a series of grid maps, recording disease events and other data for each grid cell (Astudillo, 1983; Arámbulo and Astudillo, 1991). While incorporating spatial data into the animal health information system, it is not clear whether the system incorporates any spatial analytical capability. Similarly, in Namibia, the location of all disease events is recorded, and simple disease maps are produced using spreadsheet software (Hare and Biggs, 1996). As previously mentioned, the Malaysian animal health information system incorporates the ability to map the location of disease events (Sopian Johar, pers. comm.). These systems demonstrate the acknowledged need for an understanding of the spatial distribution of disease, but have avoided the use of a fully functional GIS, probably because of the perceived expense and complexity of setting up such a system.

In Queensland, Australia, the state government has linked its animal health information system to property ownership records maintained by the Lands Department, to create the Agricultural Properties System (Baldock, 1995). Each piece of data maintained by the system is linked to the property of origin, enabling sophisticated maps and interactive queries on, for instance, chemical residues or disease diagnoses. A wide area network gives regional users real-time access to the system, via a sophisticated custom designed interface. The system is however not built on a true GIS, and therefore is not capable of more complex spatial analysis. Due to the large amount of programming effort and extensive hardware requirements, a system such as this is extremely expensive to establish. Similar systems have been established in Western Australia (Kabay and Edwards, 1997) and New Zealand (Ryan, 1997).

The potential benefits for an animal health information system are clear, but the use of powerful GIS systems (as opposed to simple disease mapping programs) seems to be limited to specific research projects and a few information systems in developed countries. This begs the question: is it feasible to incorporate a fully functional GIS into an animal health information system in a developing country, while still meeting the four criteria outlined above? That is, can GIS technology be made *cost-efficient*, *rapid*, *reliable*, and *practical* for use in animal health information systems.

2.5 Risk analysis

Because of the potential impact of infectious diseases, many countries are in the process of undertaking risk analyses to prevent the entry and spread of unwanted pathogens as trade in animal products increases under the various WTO agreements. In addition, the emergence of bovine spongiform encephalopathy (BSE) with its linkage to human health has motivated veterinary authorities to take a rigorous approach to risk analysis to avoid international spread.

For quarantine purposes, risk is defined as a combination of the likelihood of the occurrence of an undesirable event (such as an exotic disease outbreak) and the consequences of that event.

Figure 3

Risk analysis

Risk analysis incorporates the use of disease surveillance and other information to provide a scientific basis for import-export decisions. The overall framework has been outlined by Heuston (1997) and the concept is summarised in the diagram below.

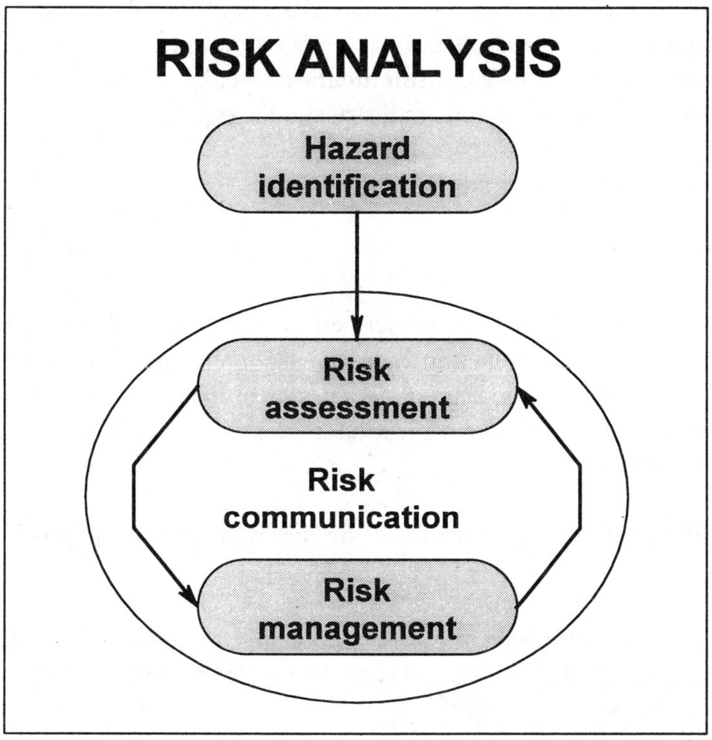

MacDiarmid (1997) has given a brief introduction to quantitative methods in risk analysis and provides a number of examples including the effects of different risk reduction measures.

Astudillo (1996) has outlined the role of risk analysis in regionalisation (creation of zones within a country of different disease status and risk). The US proposal recognises 6 levels of risk from negligible through to unknown status which is regarded as a high level of risk. Criteria have been established for each of the levels. For example, for a zone to be classified as negligible risk for a specific disease, the causal agent must not have been diagnosed during the lifetime of any currently living susceptible animal in the absence of a vaccination programme.

2.5.1 International Animal Health Code

Section 1.4 of the OIE International Animal Health Code on import risk analysis contains new concepts to be embraced by animal disease control authorities. The code consists of four chapters: General Considerations, Guidelines for Risk Assessment, Evaluation of Veterinary Services and Zoning and Regionalisation of countries.

The principle of import risk analysis is to provide importing countries with an objective, defensible method of assessing the risks associated with the importation of animals, animal products, animal genetic material, feedstuffs, biological material and pathological material. The analysis should be transparent in order that the exporting country may be provided with a clear and substantiated decision on the conditions imposed for importation or refusal for importation.

Following these principles is preferable to a zero-risk approach because it should lead to a more objective decision and enable competent authorities to discuss any differences in conclusion which may arise concerning potential risks.

The components of import risk analysis identified by the OIE include:

1. **risk assessment** (identifying and estimating the risks and evaluating the consequences), **risk management** (identification, documentation and implementation of measures that can be used to reduce the risks and their consequences) and **risk communication** (means of communicating the results of the risk assessment to decision makers, regulators, industry and the public);

2. evaluation of Competent Authorities; and

3. zoning within countries.

A standardised **risk assessment** method is prescribed in the code. The importing country should elaborate scenarios by which the introduction of a disease agent in an imported commodity and its subsequent exposure and transmission to animals is possible. Each scenario should comprise a set of factors that require identification (and quantification if possible) to allow estimation of risk. Four categories of factors are identified:

1. **Country factors**. Principally the prevalence of the disease agent in the population from which the commodity was drawn.

2. **Commodity factors**. Parameters specific to a particular commodity that affect the probability of disease agent presence and survival in a commodity at the time of import.

3. **Exposure factors**. Factors specific to the use and distribution of the commodity in the importing country which will affect the probability that a susceptible host species will be exposed and infected.

4. **Risk reduction factors**. Measures that can be applied to reduce the risk that a disease agent will be introduced into the importing country, exposed and/or transmitted to an animal.

For each of the above categories, a number of options is identified in the codes. In practice, information on each of the factors is obtained from available sources including precedents, scientific information, experience and expert opinion. Where possible, quantitative data are obtained for a factor. Where quantitative data is sparse or unreliable, a qualitative risk assessment may be made.

2.5.2 Examples of import risk analyses

In addition to an introduction to methodological concepts, a number of examples of import risk analyses are described in a recent OIE Scientific and Technical Review (OIE 1997b). Astudillo *et al* (1997) used computer simulation to make quantitative estimates of the risk of FMD virus entering the global trade of beef from some areas of South America. A risk scenario pathway comprising 6 events was developed and a range of probability estimates assigned for each event.

MacDiarmid and Thompson (1997) used a qualitative approach to examine a number of disease risks for sheep and goat meat imported into New Zealand as well as safeguards that might be required. They concluded that there were few pathogens for which specific safeguards were required, the main exception being FMD.

2.6 Computer modelling

The use of computer modelling is briefly described in this section, with bovine spongiform encephalopathy and foot and mouth disease used as examples to show the wide range of applications that have been developed. Readers are referred to more extensive texts on modelling for in-depth of principles and techniques discussions (Bailey 1975, Anderson and May 1982, Murray 1989).

In general terms, mathematical models are a set of equations which are used to describe or simulate some part of the real world (Hillier and Lieberman 1990). Three broad functions can be identified for computer models:

- to provide a systematic basis for integrating and evaluating known information about a particular system;
- to identify gaps in knowledge about a particular system;
- to assist in identifying and assessing the impact of interventions on different facets of the system.

Epidemiological models of infectious disease are extreme simplifications of complex biological systems. Despite this limitation, mathematical models are useful tools to examine theoretical disease behaviour under assumptions derived from existing knowledge. The strength of modelling is that a wide range of possible strategies to alter disease dynamics can be quickly examined at a relatively low cost. "Best bet" strategies can then be further evaluated through biological experimentation.

Mathematical modelling of infectious disease is a relatively new science and its emergence depended on the development of a general understanding of epidemic theory (Bailey 1975). Hamer (1906) was probably the first to propose that the behaviour of an epidemic depended on the number of susceptibles and the contact rate between susceptibles and infectives in a population. These basic mathematical assumptions still underpin modern epidemic theory. Today, there is a substantial body of literature on the mathematical biology of infectious diseases and quite complex models have been developed to obtain a better understanding of disease epidemics and control options such as for bovine spongiform encehpalopathy in the UK (Anderson *et al* 1996). In fact, with BSE, a relatively simple model was developed early on in the epidemic to estimate the time of onset and duration of exposure as well as the incubation period distribution and age classes of animals exposed (Wilesmith *et al* 1988). From this model, the following conclusions were made:

- both calves and adults had been exposed but the risk of exposure of calves was 30 times that of adults;
- exposure of cattle began in 1981/82 and continued to at least the end of 1984; and
- the incubation period had a range of 2.5 to 8 years and followed a log-normal distribution.

These early findings from computer modelling have been substantiated with subsequent observations as the epidemic has progressed.

To further exemplify the wide range of issues explored through modelling, foot and mouth disease will be discussed as an example. FMD modelling has been undertaken for three main purposes: to generate scenarios for economic and other follow-on analyses; to understand the population dynamics in wildlife; and to explain airborne spread. Other applications are an FMD outbreak simulation model incorporated into an epidemic management system, EpiMan (Sanson *et al* 1991b, 1993, 1997) and a model of the relationship between different vaccination strategies and herd immunity at the village level in northern Thailand (Cleland *et al* 1994).

By far the greatest use of modelling in FMD has been for economic studies (McCauley *et al* 1979, Carpenter and Thieme 1980, Thieme 1983, Dijkhuizen 1988, Dijkhuizen 1989, Young *et al* 1991, Berensten *et al* 1992). A variety of approaches to modelling an FMD epidemic have been used. For example, Miller (1979) used a state-transition approach based on a Markov chain model to simulate the size of an outbreak of FMD in the USA as part of a large study into the potential economic impact of FMD in that country (McCauley *et al* 1979). A simpler approach taken by Baldock (1993) using the Reed-Frost epidemic model (Abbey 1952, Elveback and Varma 1965) gave epidemics which behaved similarly to those of Miller (1979). Both the Miller (1979) and the Baldock (1993) models were used to generate outbreak scenarios for use in economic studies and were based on herd contact rates modified from those observed in the very extensive and well documented 1967/68 UK epidemic (Wilson 1987).

Airborne spread of FMD and other viruses occurs under certain meteorological conditions and was believed to have played a major role in the 1967/68 UK epidemic involving more than 2000 farms (Hugh-Jones and Wright 1970). Mathematical models have since been developed to analyse and predict the role of airborne spread in FMD outbreaks (Gloster *et al* 1981, Gloster *et al* 1982, Donaldson 1988). By using such models, Donaldson *et al* (1982) were able to show that outbreaks of FMD on Jersey and the Isle of Wight in 1981 probably resulted from airborne carriage across the English Channel from an outbreak in Brittany, France.

Pech and Hone (1988) used a mathematical model of the outbreak dynamics of FMD in feral pigs to study factors necessary for persistence of the virus in the population and the culling rates necessary for effective control. Pech and Hone (1988) concluded that very high culling rates would be required to eradicate FMD from feral pig populations should it become established. It is unlikely these rates could be achieved with present methods of feral pig control.

The EpiMan emergency system developed for New Zealand (Sanson *et al* 1991b, 1993, 1997) incorporates a spatial simulation model of FMD based on the actual geography of the area where the outbreak is occurring as well as data from the epidemic as it becomes available. Outputs from the model will be used to help in predicting further likely spread of the outbreak.

2.7 Methods of economic analysis

This topic has been recently reviewed by Mlangwa and Samui (1996) and will therefore not be covered in depth in this discussion. Rather, a very brief overview is given and several specific case studies described as examples of application of different methods. Mlangwa and Samui (1996) discuss the concepts, models and techniques used in animal health economics as well as demonstrate the linkages between epidemiology and economics.

Economics has an extensive theoretical apparatus and an array of methods and techniques. Animal health economics has two interrelated branches: economics for the planning and management of animal health services and economic analysis of diseases and interventions. Epidemiology and economics, although separate scientific areas, are complementary when the goal is efficient management of animal health and associated delivery systems. In performing economic analyses, an "economic model' should determine data requirements (epidemiological and socioeconomic), as such analyses invariably require epidemiological inputs.

The core concepts in economic analysis are as follows: conceptual models, opportunity cost of resources, marginal analysis and partial analysis. Important methods include statistical models, mathematical programming, budgets, cost minimisation, decision analysis, variants of cost-benefit analysis and simulation (Mlangwa and Samui 1996).

Three general examples are given below. The first concerns a general framework for economic assessment of animal health control. The second is an example of an economic assessment of the risks of introduction of an exotic disease while the third combines epidemiological and economic modelling to examine control options for infectious bovine rhinotracheitis.

Buijtels *et al* (1996) have outlined the basic framework for the economic evaluation of animal health control programmes. The further integration of international markets means that co-ordinated policies against contagious animal infections have become increasingly important, and stricter demands for control and eradication should be expected in the future. To meet these demands, it would be desirable to create a computer simulation environment in which 'what if?' scenarios could be performed, in order to explore the epidemiological and economic effects of various infections and control strategies. The authors propose a flexible economic framework and illustrate this framework with an example. The framework has four elements: changes in the percentage of infectious herds, changes in product quantities, changes in product prices and economic integration. Each element is specifically defined and has its own input and output data, depending on the control strategy under consideration. In an illustration of the framework, probability distributions of the different control strategies are compared and the optimal strategy is chosen, according to the attitude of the decision-maker towards risk. Such a framework can be considered as a new standardised approach for comparing and selecting animal health control strategies, by integrating technical and economic data and principles.

Horst *et al* (1997) have examined the risks and economic consequences of introducing classical swine fever into The Netherlands by feeding swill to swine. An effective animal disease prevention and eradication programme is of great importance for meat-exporting countries such as the Netherlands. If a serious outbreak of disease were to occur, the eradication measures required by the European Union and a possible ban on meat exports would have severe economic consequences. However, historical and experimental information on which these programmes can be based is scarce. Furthermore, until recently, an integrated approach which combined the various aspects of outbreaks and risks with economic consequences was lacking. This paper describes a project based on such an integrated approach. The project covered the elicitation of expert knowledge and the development of the virus introduction risk simulation model (VIRiS). VIRiS integrates objective and subjective information concerning risks and consequences of virus introduction, and thus presents policy-makers with a useful tool for the evaluation of existing prevention programmes and possible alternatives. VIRiS is illustrated for classical swine fever. A comparison is made between the current situation and a hypothetical situation where the risk factor 'swill feeding' is completely eliminated.

Vonk Noordegraaf *et al* (1998) developed an epidemiological and economic simulation model to evaluate the spread and control of infectious bovine rhinotracheitis in The Netherlands. Bovine herpesvirus type I (BHV1), causing infectious bovine rhinotracheitis (IBR), was introduced in the Netherlands in 1971. In 1993, about 42% of the dairy cows had antibodies against BHV1. In the future, stricter requirements are anticipated regarding the health status of exported breeding cows and material. To support policymakers in their decisions on IBR eradication, a simulation model was developed in which the epidemiological and economic consequences of various control strategies were evaluated. In the model, dairy herds were classified into different disease states based on (1) the reproduction ratio of the disease (R, defined as the number of secondary cases caused by one infectious animal) (2) the within-herd prevalence, within each value of R and (3) the expected number of infectious animals in an infectious herd within each prevalence range. The dynamic transition probability of a herd going from one state to another per week depends on direct contacts between animals, and other contacts such as transmission through fomites, indirect transmission through other species, airborne transmission and minor disease-specific routes such as venereal or iatrogenic transmission. Five control strategies, including both a voluntary vaccination program and a compulsory vaccination program for all dairy herds were evaluated. A voluntary vaccination program with 50% participation is not expected to lead to eradication of IBR. It appears that compulsory vaccination would be necessary to reach an IBR-free status.

References and further reading

Abbey II. 1952. An examination of the Reed-Frost theory of epidemics. *HumanBiology* **24**: 201-233.

Abila RC. 1997. The Philippines animal health information system. Proceedings, Epidemiology Program, 10th FAVA Congress, Cairns Australia. pp 127-130.

Abila RC, Joco LM. in press. Country Report - Philippines. In: Sharma P. (ed) *Proceedings of the International Workshop on a Regional Computerised Animal Health Information System, June 3-5, 1997, Vientiane, Lao PDR.* Australian Centre for International Agricultural Research, Canberra.

Alderink FL. 1985. The national animal disease surveillance program: Determining the cost of livestock disease. *Journal of Veterinary Medical Education* **2**:109-110

Anderson RK. 1982. Surveillance: criteria for evaluation and design of epidemiologic surveillance systems for animal health and productivity. In: *Proceedings of 86th Annual Meeting of the United States Animal Health Association, Nashville, Tennessee, November, 1982.* United States Animal Health Association, Richmond, pp 321-341.

Anderson RM, Donnelly CA, Ferguson NM, *et al.* 1996. Transmission dynamics and epidemiology of BSE in British cattle. *Nature* **382**: 779-788.

Anderson RM, May RM (Editors). 1982. *Population Biology of Infectious Diseases.* Springer Verlag, Berlin. 314 pp

Andrews L. 1988. Animal health information systems in Australia. *Revue Scientifique et Technical d'Office International des Epizooties* 7:569-575

Anker M. 1991. Epidemiological and statistical methods for rapid health assessment. Introduction. *World Health Statistics Quarterly* **44**:94-97

Anon. 1990a. Improvement of animal disease reporting in the Asian and Pacific region. Vol I: The proceedings of a regional workshop on animal disease reporting. Asian Development Bank and Office International Epizooties, 186 pp.

Anon. 1990b. Improvement of animal disease reporting in the Asian and Pacific region. Vol II: A review of country needs and potentials for international collaboration. Asian Development Bank and Office International Epizooties, 160 pp.

Anon. 1990. *Guide to epidemiological surveillance for rinderpest.* Office International des Ipizooties, Paris

Astudillo VM. 1983. Information and surveillance system of vesicular diseases in the Americas. Use of grid maps for monitoring data collection and reporting. *Revue Scientifique et Technical d'Office International des Epizooties* **2**:739-749

Astudillo VM. 1996. The role of Risk Analysis in Regionalization. *Bulletin of the OIE.* pp 125-132.
Astidillo VM, Sutmoller P, Saraiva V, López A. 1997. Rishs of introducing foot and mouth disease through the importation of beef from South America. *Rev. sci. tech. Off. int Epiz.* **16**: 33-44

Arámbulo III PV, Astudillo V. 1991. Perspectives on the application of remote sensing and geographic information system to disease control and health management. *Prev. Vet. Med.* **11**: 345-352.

Bailey NTJ. 1975. The mathematical theory of infectious diseases - second edition. Charles Griffin and Co Ltd, London. 413 pp.

Baldock FC, Garner MG. 1998. Australia's national animal health information system. Proceedings, XX World Buriatrics Congress, Sydney Australia. pp 31-35

Baldock FC. 1993. The use of mathematical modelling in understanding foot and mouth disease. In: Nunn MJ, Thornber PM. Proceedings of the national symposium on foot and mouth disease. Australian Government Publishing Service. pp 177-190.

Baldock FC. 1995. A Queensland response to changing information needs in animal health. In: Morton J. (ed) *Epidemiology Chapter, Australian College of Veterinary Scientists Proceedings. Australian Veterinary Association Annual Conference, Melbourne, May 21-26, 1995.* Australian College of Veterinary Scientists, Indooroopilly, pp 54-59.

Beal VC Jr. 1983. Perspectives on animal disease surveillance. In: *Proceedings of the 87th Annual Meeting of United States Animal Health Association, October, 1983.* United States Animal Health Association, Richmond

Bedard BG, McClure LH, Akoso BT. 1991. The epidemiological function of diagnostic laboratories in developing countries. In: Martin SW. (ed) *Proceedings of the 6th International Society for Veterniary Epidemiolgy and Economics symposium, Ottawa, Canada, 12-16 August, 1991.* University of Guelph, Ontario, pp 196-200.

Bedard BG, Hutabarat TSP, Johar S, Meephuch Y, Joco MLM. 1997. Animal health and production information system Proceedings, Epidemiology Program, 10th FAVA Congress, Cairns Australia. pp 115-121.

Belfrage JB, Salman MD, Freier J, Nuckols J, Otto D. 1994. A geographic information system analysis of pseudorabies (Aujesky's disease) in four counties in Iowa, USA. *Ken. Vet.* **18**: 500.

Bennett S, Woods T, Liyanage WM, Smith DL. 1991. A simplified general method for cluster-sample surveys of health in developing countries. *World Health Statistics Quarterly* **44**:98-106

Bernardo TM, Schotman C, Stemshorn BW, Waltner-Toews D. 1991. The Caribbean animal and plant health information network (CARAPHIN): information related to trade. In: Martin SW. (ed) *Proceedings of the 6th International Symposium on Veterinary Epidemiology and Economics, Ottawa, Canada, 12-16 August, 1991.* University of Guelph, Ontario, pp 193-195.

Berensten PBM, Dijkhuizen AA, Oskam AJ. 1992. A dynamic model for cost-benefit analyses of foot and mouth disease control strategies. *Preventive Veterinary Medicine* **12**: 229-243.

Bertrand EW. 1985. Microcomputer applications in health population surveys: experience and potential in developing countries. *World Health Statistics Quarterly* **38**:91-99

Biggs HC, Hare KM. 1994. Essential features of an integrated veterinary disease information system for Namibia. *The Kenya Veterinarian* **18**:29-31

Birkett NJ. 1988. Computer-aided personal interviewing. A new technique for data collection in epidemiologic surveys. *American Journal of Epidemiology* **127**:684-690

Black P, Pitt D, Ward M, Mackenzie A, Cronin J, Baldock C. 1997. The implementation of an active animal health surveillance program for the beef industry of Queensland, Australia. Proceedings, Epidemiology Program, 10th FAVA Congress, Cairns Australia. pp 139-146.

Blajan L. 1979. The systems for veterinary information at the national and world-wide levels. Bulletin of the OIE **91**: 795-821.

Blajan L, Chillaud T. 1991. The OIE world animal disease information system. *Revue Scientifique et Technical d'Office International des Epizooties* **10**:71-87

Blood DC, Brightling P. 1988. National Animal Disease Databanks. In: Veterinary Information Management. Bailliere Tindall, London. pp 153-160.

Buijtels JA, Huirne RB, Dijkhuizen AA, Renkema JA, Noordhuizen JP. 1996. Basic framework for the economic evaluation of animal health control programmes. *Rev Sci Tech* **15**(3):775-95.

Cameron A. 1997. Using geographical information systems in livestock disease control. Proceedings, Epidemiology Program, 10th FAVA Congress, Cairns Australia. pp 177-184.

Cameron AR, Baldock FC. 1998a. A new probability formula for surveys to substantiate freedom from disease. *Preventive Veterinary Medicine* **34**: 1-17.

Cameron AR, Baldock FC. 1998b. Two-stage sampling to substantiate freedom from disease. *Preventive Veterinary Medicine* **34**: 19-30.

Campbell CL. 1989. *Geographical information system applications in animal health.* 47-62.

Cannon RM. 1993. ANADIS: Monitoring the eradication of brucellosis and tuberculosis in Australia. *Agricultural Systems and Information Technology* **5**:11-13

Cannon RM, Roe RT. 1982. Livestock disease surveys - a field manual for veterinarians. Aust Gov Publ Service, Canberra. 35 pp.

Carpenter TE, Thieme A. 1980. A simulation approach to measuring the economic effects of foot and mouth disease in beef and dairy cattle. Proceedings 2nd International Symposium on Veterinary Epidemiology and Economics pp 511-516

Chaisrisongkram W. 1994. An overview of foot-and-mouth disease control in Thailand. In: Copland JW, Gleeson LJ, Chamnanpood C. (eds) *ACIAR Proceedings No. 51: Diagnosis and epidemiology of foot-and-mouth disease in Southeast Asia. Proceedings of an international workshop held at Lampang, Thailand, September 6-9, 1993.* Australian Centre for International Agricultural Research, Canberra, pp 23-25.

Chambers R, Pacey A, Thrupp LA. (eds) (1989) *Farmer First: Farmer Innovation and Agricultural Research.* Intermediate Technology Publications, London

Chillaud T. 1997. Information requirements, including OIE specifications. Proceedings, Epidemiology Program, 10th FAVA Congress, Cairns Australia. pp 109-114.

Chrea S, Chhoeung B. in press. Country Report - Kingdom of Combodia. In: Sharma P. (ed) *Proceedings of the International Workshop on a Regional Computerised Animal Health Information System, June 3-5 1997, Vientiane, Loa PDR.* Australian Centre for International Agriculture Research, Canberra.

CIA. 1997. *CIA World Factbook, 1996 (Internet edition)* http://www.odci.gov/cia/publications/pubs.html

Cleland PC, Baldock FC, Gleeson LJ, Chamnanpood P. 1994. A modelling approach to the investigation of vaccination strategies for foot and mouth disease in Thailand. (Proc 7th Int Symp Vet Epidemiol and Econ, Nairobi) Kenya Vet **18**: 394-397.

Cochran WG. 1977. *Sampling Techniques.* 3rd ed. John Wiley and Sons Inc. New York.

Dahl J. 1985. NADS: implications for the livestock industry. *Journal of Veterinary Medical Education.* **2:** 112.

Dale PE, Ritchie SA, Territo BM, Morris CD, Muhar A, Kay BH. 1998. An overview of remote sensing and GIS for surveillance of mosquito vector habitats and risk assessment. *Journal Vector Ecology* **23**: 54-61

Davies FG, Kilelu E, Linthicum KJ, Pegram RG. 1992. Patterns of Rift Valley fever activity in Zambia. *Epidemiology and Infection* **108**: 185 191.

Diesch SL. 1988. Development and application of animal health information systems. In: *Environment and Animal Health: Proceedings of the 6th International Congress I n Animal Hygiene, Skara, Sweden, 14-17 June, 1988* pp 185-189.

Dijkhuizen AA. 1988. Epidemiological and economic evaluation of foot and mouth disease control strategies using a Markov chain spreadsheet model. Proceedings 5th International Symposium on Veterinary Epidemiology and Economics pp 350-352.

Dijkhuizen AA. 1989. Epidemiological and economic evaluation of foot and mouth disease control strategies in the Netherlands. *Netherlands Journal Agricultural Science* **37**: 1-12.

Dister SW, Fish D, Bros SM, Frank DH, Wood BL. 1997. Landscape characterization of peridomestic risk for Lyme disease using satellite imagery. *American Journal Tropical Medicine and Hygiene* **57**: 687-692.

Donaldson AI. 1988. Development and use of models for forecasting the airborne spread of foot and mouth disease. *Journal of the Royal Agricultural Society of England* **149**: 184-194.

Donaldson AI, Gloster J, Harvey LDJ, Deans DH. 1982. Use of prediction models to forecast and analyse airborne spread during the foot and mouth disease outbreaks in Brittany, Jersey and the Isle of Wight in 1981. *Veterinary Record* **110**: 53-57.

Doohoo IR. 1988. Animal Productivity and Health Information Network. *Canadian Veterinary Journal* **29**: 281-287.

Eleveback L, Varma A. 1965. Simulation of mathematical models for public health problems. *Public Health Reports* **80**: 1067-1076.

Ellis PR. 1994. Information systems in disease control programs. In: Copland JW, Gleeson LJ, Chamnonpood C. (eds) *ACIAR Proceedings No. 51: Diagnosis and epidemiology of foot and mouth disease in Southeast Asia. Proceedings of an international workshop help at Lampang, Thailand September 6-9 1993.* Australian Centre for International Agricultural Research, Canberra, pp 111-115

English D. 1992. Geographical epidemiology and ecological studies. In: Elliot P, Cuzick J, English D, Stern R. (eds) *Geographical and Environmental Epidemiology. Methods for small-area studies.* Oxford University Press, Oxford, Published on behalf of the WHO Regional Office for Europe, pp 3-13.

Estrada-Pena A. 1999. Geostatistics and remote sensing using NOAA-AVHRR satellite imagery as predictive tools in tick distribution and habitat suitability estimations for Boophilus microplus (Acari: Ixodidae) in South America. National Oceanographic and Atmosphere Administration-Advanced Very High Resolution Radiometer. *Veterinary Parasitology* **81**: 73-82.

Ezeokoli CD, Obi TU, Majiyagbe KA. 1990. Sero-monitoring the Nigerian national herd for rinderpest. In: *The sero-monitoring of rinderpest throughout Africa. Phase One. Proceedings of a Final Research Co-ordination Meeting of the FAO/IAEA/SIDA/OAU/IBAR/PARC Coordinated Research Programme, Bingerville, Cote d'Ivoire, 19-23 November, 1990.* International Atomic Energy Agency (IAEA), Vienna, pp 187-200.

FAO/IAEA. 1993. Recommended Procedures for Disease and Serological Surveillance as part of the Global Rinderpest Eradication Programme - GREP. 51 pp.

Farrar J. 1988. The National Animal Heatlh Monitoring System (NAHMS): Progression from a pilot project to a national program. In: *Proceedings of the 6th International Symposium on Veterinary Epidemiology and Economics, Copenhagen, Denmark, 1988.* International Society for Veterinary Epidemiology and Economics (ISVEE), Copenhagen, 191-193.

Faugère O, Merlin P, Faugère B. 1991. Evaluation of health and productivity of small ruminants in Africa: the example of Sengal. *Revue Scientifique et Technical d'Office International des Epizooties* **10**: 131-150

Flasse S, Walker C, Biggs H, Stephenson P, Hutchinson P. 1998. Using remote sensing to predict outbreaks of Oestrus ovis in Namibia. *Preventive Veterinary Medicine* **33**: 31-38.

Forman AJ, Leslie J. 1997.*Foot and Mouth Disease Surveillance, Control and Strategy Formulation. Report of the Technical Assessment Mission, January/February, 1997.* Food and Agriculture Organisation (FAO), Bangkok (TCP/RAS/6611 Field Document No. 3)

Frerichs RR. 1989. Simple analytic procedures for rapid microcomputer-assisted cluster surveys in developing countries. *Public Health Reports* **104**:24-35

Frerichs RR, Tar Tar K. 1989. Computer-assisted rapid surveys in developing countries. *Public Health Reports* **104**:14-23

Gardner I. 1990. Reporting disease outbreaks. In: Epidemiology at work. Proc 144, Post Graduate Committee in Veterinary Science, University of Sydney pp 29-42.

Garner MG, Nunn MJ. 1991. Requirements for an Australian Animal Health Information System. In: Sergeant, E.S.G. (ed) *Epidemiology Chapter Proceedings, AVA/NZVA Pan Pacific Conference on Veterinarians and the Environment, Sydney, May, 1991*. Australian College of Veterinary Scientists, Sydney, 7-16.

Garner MG. 1993. A national animal health information system for Australia. *Agricultural Systems and Information Technology* **5**:9-11

Garner MG. 1997. The Australian National Animal Health Informtion System. In: More S. (ed) *Proceedings of the Epidemiology Program, 10th FAVA Congress, Cairns, 24th - 28th August, 1997*. University of Queensland, Brisbane, 147-156

Glosser JW. 1988. Back to the future: The animal health monitoring system - a political necessity being addressed in the United States. In: *Proceedings of the 5th International Symposium on Veterinary Epidemiology and Economics, Copenhagen, Denmark, 1988*. International Society for Veterinary Epidemiology and Economics, Copenhagen, 42-48

Gloster J, Blackall RM, Sellers RF, Donaldson AI. 1981. Forecasting the airborne spread of foot and mouth disease. *Veterinary Record* **108**: 370-374.

Gloster J, Sellers RF, Donaldson AI. 1982. Long distance transport of foot and mouth disease virus over the sea. *Veterinary Record* **110**: 47-52

Hanyanum W, Awaiyawanon K, Wongdee R, Musikul P. 1994. Thailand. In: Copland JW, Gleeson LJ, Chamnanpood C. (eds) *ACIAR Proceedings No. 51: Diagnosis and epidemiology of foot-and-mouth disease in Southeast Asia. Proceedings of an international workshop held at Lampang, Thailand, September 6-9, 1993*. Australian Centre for International Agricultural Research, Canberra pp 191-196.

Hamer WH. 1906. Epidemic disease in England. *Lancet* **1**: 733-739.

Hare KM, Biggs HC. 1996. Design and evaluation of a veterinary information system for Namibia. *Preventive Veterinary Medicine* **26**: 239-251.

Harris DR, Lemeshow S. 1991. Evaluation of the EPI survey methodology for estimating relative risk. *World Health Statistics Quarterly* **44**:107-114

Hassan AN, Beck LR, Dister S. 1998. Prediction of villages at risk for filariasis transmission in the Nile Delta using remote sensing and geographic information system technologies. *Journal Egyptian Society Parasitology* **28**: 75-87

Hay SI, Snow RW, Rogers DJ. 1998. Predicting malaria seasons in Kenya using multitemporal meteorological satellite sensor data. *Transactions Royal Society Tropical Medicine and Hygiene* **92**: 12-20.

Henderson RH, Sundaresan T. 1982. Cluster sampling to assess immunization coverage: a review of experience with a simplified sampling method. *Bulletin of the World Health Organisation* **60**: 253-260

Hoffsis GF. 1985. The national animal diseasesurveillance program: Implications for the veterinary practitioner. *Journal of Veterinary Medical Education.* **2**:111

Hueston WD. 1993. Assessment of national systems for the surveillance and monitoring of animal disease. *Revue Scientifique et Technical d'Office International des Epizooties* **12**:1187-1196

Heuston WD. 1997. Risk analysis. Proceedings, 8th International Symposium on Veterinary Epidemiology and Economics, Paris. pp viii-x.

Horst HS, Huirne RB, Dijkhuizen AA. 1997. Risks and economic consequences of introducing classical swine fever into The Netherlands by feeding swill to swine. *Rev Sci Tech* **16**(1):207-14.

Hugh-Jones M. 1991a. Introductory remarks on the application of remote sensing and geographic information systems to epidemiology and disease control. *Prev. Vet. Med.* **11**: 159-161.

Hugh-Jones M. 1991b. Satellite imaging as a technique for obtaining disease-related data. *Rev. Sci. Tech. Off. Int. Epi.* **10**: 197-204.

Hugh-Jones M.E. 1993. Applying remote sensing and geographic information systems to epidemiology and disease control. *Agricultural Systems and Information Technology* **5**: 6-8.

Hugh-Jones ME, Wright PB. 1970. Studies on the 1967-8 foot and mouth disease epidemic (The relation of weather to the spread of disease). *Journal of Hygiene, Cambridge* **68**: 253-271.

Hugh-Jones ME, O'Niel P. 1985. *The epidemiological uses of remote sensing and satellites.* Proceedings of the 4th International Symposium on Veterinary Epidemiology & Economics, 18-22 November 1985, Singapore. pp 113-118.

Hurd HS, Hancock DD, Thomas LA, Wells SJ. 1994. Salmonella prevalence in US dairy calves and a comparison of active and passive surveillance systems. In: *Proceedings of the VIIIth Congress of the International Society for Animal Hygiene, St Paul, Minnesota.* International Society for Animal Hygiene, St Paul

Hutabarat TSPN, Morris RS. 1997. The development of an animal health information system for Indonesia. Proceedings, Epidemiology Program, 10th FAVA Congress, Cairns Australia. pp 131-138.

IAEA (1992) The sero-monitoring of rinderpest throughout Africa. Phase II. Results for 1992. In: *Proceedings of a Research Co-ordination Meeting of the FAO/IAEA/SIDA/OAU/IBAR/PARC Coordinated Research Programme, Entebbe, Uganda, 15-21 September, 1992*

Jordan D. 1995. Aggregate testing for the evaluation of Johne's disease herd status. In: Morton J (Ed), Epidemiology Chapter, Australian College of Veterinary Scientists Proceedings. Australian Veterinary Association Annual Conference, Melbourne, May 21-26, 1995. Australian College of Veterinary Scientists, Indooroopilly. pp 60-67.

Kabay MJ, Edwards JR. 1997. Information technology for industry resource protection in Western Australia. In: More, S. (ed) *Proceedings of the Epidemiology Program, 10th FAVA Congress, Cairns, 24th - 28th August, 1997.* University of Queensland, Brisbane, pp 161-165.

Kadir I, Johar S, Nordin Nor M. 1997. Malaysia animal health information system. In: More, S. (ed) *Proceedings of the Epidemiology Program, 10th FAVA Congress, Cairns, 24th - 28th August, 1997.* University of Queensland, Brisbane, Supplementary Paper.

Kelch WJ, New JC Jr. 1993. The reported use of drugs to prevent diseases in beef cattle in Tennessee. *Preventive Veterinary Medicine* **15**:291-302

Kellar JA. The effect of infrastructure on surveillance and monitoring programs. 1996. Comprehensive reports on technical items presented to the International Committee or to Regional Commissions. OIE, Paris. pp 125-132.

King LJ. 1985. Unique characteristics of the national animal disease surveillance system. *Journal of the American Veterinary Medical Association* **186**: 35-39.

King LJ. 1988. National Animal Health Monitoring System in the USA: a model information system for international animal health. *Revue Scientifique et Technical d'Office International des Epizooties* 7:583-588

King LJ. 1994. Office of international épizooties (OIE) strategies for international animal health information systems. *The Kenya Veterinarian* **18**:47-47

King LJ. 1986. The National Animal Health Monitoring System (NAHMS): an early assessment. In: *Proceedings of 90th Annual Meeting of the United States Animal Health Association, Louisville, Kentucky, October 19-24, 1986*. United States Animal Health Association, Richmond, pp 86-91.

Kish L. 1995. *Survey Sampling.* John Wiley and Sons, New York.

Kitron U. 1998. Landscape ecology and epidemiology of vector-borne diseases: tools for spatial analysis. *Journal Medical Entomology* **35**: 435-445.

Lai Thi Kim L, Thai Thi Thuy P. in press. Country Report - Vietnam. In: Sharma P. (ed) *Proceedings of the International Workshop on a Regional Computerised Animal Health Information System, June 3-5, 1997, Vientiane, Lao PDR.* Australian Centre for International Agricultural Research, Canberra.

Last, J.M. (ed) (1988) *A Dictionary of Epidemiology*, 2nd ed. Oxford University Press, New York.

Lemeshow S, Robinson D. 1985. Surveys to measure programme coverage and impact: a review of the methodology used by the expanded programme on immunization. *World Health Statistics Quarterly* **38**:65-75

Lessard P, l'Eplattenier R, Norval RAI, Perry BD, Dolan TT, Burrill A, Croze H, Sorensen M, Grootenhuis JG, Irvin AD. 1988. The use of geographical information systems in estimating east coast fever risk to African livestock. *Acta. Vet. Scand.*:234-236

Lessard PR, Perry BD. 1988. Investigation of disease outbreaks and impaired productivity. *The Veterinary Clinics of North America, Food Animal Practice.* Vol 4, Number 1.

Levaro JV, Guillen BJ. 1983. *Animal disease reporting in Mexico.* Proceedings of the 87th Annual Meeting of United States Animal Health Association, October, 1983.

Levy PS, Lemeshow S. 1991. *Sampling of Populations: Methods and Applications*, 2nd ed. John Wiley & Sons, Inc, New York.

Linthicum KJ, Bailey CL, Tucker CJ, Mitchell KD, Logan TM, Davies FG, Kamau CW, Thande PC, Wagateh JN. 1990. Application of polar-orbiting, meteorological satellite data to detect flooding of Rift Valley Fever virus vector mosquito habitats in Kenya. Medical and Veterinary Entomology **4**: 433-438

Lossinger WC, Bush EJ, Hill GW, Smith MA, Garber LP, Rodriguez JM, Kane G. 1998. Design and implementation of the United States National Animal Health Monitoring System 1995 National Swine Study. *Preventive Veterinary Medicine* **34**: 147-159.

McCauley EH, New Jr JC, Aulaqi NA, Sundquist WB, Miller WM (eds). 1979. A study of the potential economic impact of foot-and-mouth disease in the United States. Univ Minnesota, St Paul MA. 240 pp

MacDiarmid SC. 1997. Risk analysis and the international trade in animals and their products. In: Dijkhuizen AA, Morris RS (Eds). *Animal Health Economics - Principles and Applications. Post Graduate Foundation in Veterinary Science*, University of Sydney. 306 pp.

MacDiarmid SC, Thompson EJ. 1997. The potential risks to animal health from imported sheep and goat meat. *Rev. sci. tech. Off. Int. Epiz.* **16:** 45-56

Marsh WE, Damrongwatanapokin T, Larntz K, Morrison RB. 1991a. The use of a geographic information system in an epidemiological study of pseudorabies (Aujeszky's disease) in Minnesota swine herds. *Prev. Vet. Med.* **11**: 249-254.

Marsh WE, Damrongwatanapokin T, Morrison RB, Larntz K., Anderson PL, Bearman J. 1991b. Application of a geographic information system to identify risk factors for infectious diseases of swine. In: Martin, S.W. (ed)

Proceedings of the 6th ISVEE symposium, Ottawa, Canada, 12-16 August, 1991. University of Guelph, Ontario. pp 535-537.

Martin FB. 1983. Statistical practice in the NADS pilot studies. In: *Proceedings of the 87th Annual Meeting of United States Animal Health Association, October, 1983.* United States Animal Health Association, Richmond.

Martin SW, Meek AH, Willeberg P. 1987. Veterinary epidemiology - principles and methods. Iowa State Univ Press, Ames Iowa. pp 283-291.

Martinez TA, Kaneene JB, Lloyd JW, Brown MI. 1992. Potential users and user requirements of an animal-health monitoring system in a developing country: case study of Honduras. *Preventive Veterinary Medicine* **13**: 1-11.

Mayer D, Atzeni M. 1993. Invasion of the dreaded screw-worm fly: Prediction of economic consequences and control strategies. *Agricultural Systems and Information Technology* **5**: 22-24.

McCallon WR, Beal VC Jr. 1982a. The fallacy of drawing inferences from biased data: some case examples. In: *Proceedings of the 86th Annual Meeting of United States Animal Health Association.* United States Animal Health Association, Richmond, pp 350-358.

McCallon WR, Beal VC Jr. 1982b. Historical aspects of animal disease reporting and the development of a national animal disease surveillance system. In: *Proceedings of 86th Annual Meeting of United States Animal Health Association, Northville, USA, November 7-12, 1982.* United States Animal Health Association, Richmond, pp 341-349.

McGinn TJ III, Wray DW, Cowen P. 1994. Medical geography of Aujesky's disease in North Carolina, USA: the effect of density of swine and prevalence of infection on a neighbouring Aujesky's disease status. *The Kenya Veterinarian* **18**:499

McKenzie J, Thompson J. 1991. New Zealand's national animal health information system. *Surveillance* **18**: 12-15.

Meephuch Y. 1994. An information system developed for monitoring foot-and-mouth disease control in Thailand. In: Copland JW, Gleeson LJ, Chamnanpood C. (eds) *ACIAR Proceedings No. 51: Diagnosis and epidemiology of foot-and-mouth disease in Southeast Asia. Proceedings of an international workshop held at Lampang, Thailand, September 6-9, 1993.* Australian Centre for International Agricultural Research, Canberra, pp 116-118

Meephuch Y. in press. Country Report - Thailand. In: Sharma, P. (ed) *Proceedings of the International Workshop on a Regional Computerised Animal Health Information System, June 3-5, 1997, Vientiane, Lao PDR.* Australian Centre for International Agricultural Research, Canberra

Meier HP, Hauser R. 1996. The monitoring of infections diseases in Switzerland. *Pferdeheikunde* **12**: 569-570.

Mekhagnomdara S. 1996. *Country Report of Lao PDR.* Second Meeting of the OIE Sub-commission forFMD in South-East Asia, Vientiane, 27 February - 1 March, 1996

Mekhagnomdara S, Vongthilath S. 1994. Laos. In: Copland JW, Gleeson LJ, Chamnanpood C. (eds) *ACIAR Proceedings No. 51: Diagnosis and epidemiology of foot-and-mouth disease in Southeast Asia. Proceedings of an international workshop held at Lampang, Thailand, September 6- 9, 1993.* Australian Centre for International Agricultural Research, Canberra, pp150-154.

Mikkelsen B. 1995. *Methods for development work and research - A guide for practitioners.* Sage, London.

Miller WM. 1979. A state-transition model for epidemic foot-and-mouth disease. In: McCauley EH, New Jr JC, Aulaqi NA, Sundquist WB, Miller WM (eds). A study of the potential economic impact of foot-and-mouth disease in the United States. Univ Minnesota, St Paul MA. pp 113-131.

Mlangwa JE, Samui KL. 1996. The nature of animal health economics in relation to veterinary epidemiology. *Rev Sci Tech* **15**(3):797-812.

Morley RS. 1988. National Animal Health Information System, Agriculture Canada. *Revue Scientifique et Technical d'Office International des Epizooties* **7**: 577-581

Morris RS. 1991. Information systems for animal health: objectives and components. Rev sci tech Off int Epiz **10**: 13-23.

Morris RS. 1976. Animal health information systems. In: Ellis PR, Shaw APM, Stephens AJ. (eds) *New Techniques in Veterinary Epidemiology and Economics. Proceedings of an International Symposium held at the University of Reading, England, July, 1976.* Reading, 1976

Mulhern, F.J., (1985) The national animal disease surveillance program: International implications. *Journal of Veterinary Medical Education* **2**:113-114

Murray JD. 1989. *Mathematical Biology*. Springer Verlag, Berlin. 745 pp.

Norman HS, Sischo WM, Day RL, Pitcher P, Nesselrodt A. 1994. Evaluating the influence of neighbouring swine herd status on the spread of pseudorabies virus using a geographical information system. *Ken. Vet.* **18**: 490-492.

Nuttall I, Rumisha DW, Pilatwe TRK, Ali HI, Mokgweetsinyana SS, Sylla AH, Talla I. 1994. GIS management tools for the control of tropical diseases:Applications in Botswana, Senegal and Morocco. In: De Savigny D, Wijeyaratne P. (eds) *GIS for Health and the Environment. Proceedings of an International Workshop, Colombo, Sri Lanka, 5-10 September, 1994.* International Development Research Centre, Ottawa, pp 59-73.

Oka M, Widowati N, Lubis N, Holden S. 1992. The role of laboratory and veterinary diagnosis in Indonesia's National Disease Surveillance System. In: Daniels PW, Holden S, Lewin E, Dadi S. (eds) *Livestock Services for Smallholders: a critical evaluation of the delivery of animal health and production services to the small-scale farmer in the developing world. Proceedings of an International Seminar held at Yogyakarta, Indonesia, 15-21 November, 1992.* Directorate General of Livestock
Services, Indonesia, Yogyakarta, pp 56-59

Ogundipe GAT, Oluokun SB, Esuruoso GO. 1989. The development and efficiency of the animal health information system in Nigeria. *Preventive Veterinary Medicnine* 7: 121-135.

Ogwang F, Heinonen R. 1994. Computerised district reporting (CDR) with help of a geographical information system for veterinary services in Uganda. *Ken. Vet.* **18**: 58-60.

OIE. 1988. Veterinary Information Systems. Rev sci tech Off int Epiz **7**: 439-638.

OIE. 1991. Epidemiological Systems. Rev sci tech Off int Epiz **10**: 7-231.

OIE (1992) *World Animal Health in 1992.* Office International des Épizooties, Paris

OIE. 1997a. Recommended standards for epidemiological surveillance systems for contagious bovine pleuropneumonia. 10 pp.

OIE. 1997b. Contamination of animal health products: prevention and risks for animal health. Rev sci tech Off int Epiz Vol 16, 284 pp.

OIE. 1998. Recommended standards for epidemiological surveillance systems for rinderpest. 6 pp.

OIE and WHO. 1994. *The Marrakesh Agreement Establishing the World Trade Organisation including the Agreement on the Application of Sanitary and Phytosanitary Measure, signed in Marrakesh on 15 April, 1994 and the role assigned to the Office International des Epizooties.*

Oranga HM. 1994. A GIS approach to the determination of catchment populations around local health facilities in developing countries. In: De Savigny D, Wijeyaratne P (eds) *GIS for Health and the Environment. Proceedings of an International Workshop, Colombo, Sri Lanka, 5-10 September, 1994.* International

Development Research Centre, Ottawa. pp 53-57.

Paling RW, Leak SG, Katende J, Kamunya G, Moloo SK. 1987. Epidemiology of animal trypanosomiasis on a cattle ranch in Kilifi, Kenya. *Acta Trop* **44**: 67-82.

Pech RP, Hone J. 1988. A model of the dynamics and control of an outbreak of foot and mouth disease in feral pigs in Australia. *Journal of Applied Ecology* **25**: 63-77.

Perry BD, Norval RAI, Kruska RL, Ushewokunze-Obatolu U, Booth TH. 1991. Predicting the epidemiology of tick-borne diseases of cattle in Zimbabwe using geographic information systems. In: Martin, S.W. (ed) *Proceedings of the 6th ISVEE symposium, Ottawa, Canada, 12-16 August, 1991*. University of Guelph, Ontario. pp 214-216.

Pfeiffer DU, and Morris, RS. 1994. Spatial analysis techniques in veterinary epidemiology. *The Kenya Veterinarian* **18**:483-485

Pfeiffer DU, Morris RS, Harris A, Jackson R, Paterson B. 1991. The epidemiology of Bovine Tuberculosis in the Common Brushtail Possum. In: Martin SW. (ed) *Proceedings of the 6th International Symposium on Veterinary Epidemiology and Economics, Ottawa, Canada, 12-16 August 1991*. ISVEE, Guelph, Ontario, Canada. pp 430-433.

Pharo HJ. 1997. Using surveillance information for risk analysis and assessment for planning of disease control programs. Proceedings, Epidemiology Program, 10th FAVA Congress, Cairns Australia. pp 185-188.Ramsay GC, Black PF, Baldock FC. 1995. Assessing herd status for infectious disease using abattoir sampling. In: Morton J. (ed) *Epodemiology Chapter, Australian College of veterinary Scientists Proceedings. Australian Veterinary Association Annual conference, Melbourne, May 21-26, 1995.* Australian College of Veterinary Scientists, Indooroopilly, pp 68-70.

Poppensiek GC. 1985. The national animal disease surveillance program: a new concept. *Journal of Veterinary Medical Education* **2**:104-105.

Queensland Department of Primary Industries (1995) *Structured Animal Health Surveillance - 1994.* Queensland Department of Primary Industries, Central Region

Robertson ID, and Blackmore DK. 1985. *Abattoir data as a source of epidemiological information: a neglected resource.* Proceedings of the 4th International Symposium on Veterinary Epidemiology and Economics, 18-22 November 1985, Singapore pp 377-381.

Rogers DJ, Williams BG. 1993. Monitoring trypanosomiasis in space and time. *Parasitology* **106**: S77-S92.

Rolfe DC. 1985. Disease Information Systems. Proc No 79, Post-Graduate Committee in Veterinary Science, Univ Sydney. pp 87-112.

Rolfe DC. 1985. The development of an animal disease information system. In: *Proceedings of the 4th International Symposium on Veterinary Epidemiology & Economics, Singapore, 18-22 November, 1985.* International Society for Veterinary Epidemiology and Economics (ISVEE), Singapore, 362-364

Ryan T. 1997. The National Livestock Database in New Zealand. In: More, S. (ed) *Proceedings of the Epidemilogy Program, 10th FAVA Congress, Cairns, 24th - 28th August, 1997.* University of Queensland, Brisbane, pp 167-170.

Sanson RL, Pfeiffer DU, Morris RS. 1991a. Geographic information systems: their application in animal disease control. *Rev. Sci. Tech. Off. Int. Epi.* **10**: 179-195.

Sanson RL, Liberona H, Morris RS. 1991b. The use of a geographical information system in the management of a foot-and-mouth disease epidemic. *Preventive Veterinary Medicine* **11**:309-313

Sanson RL, Morris RS, Stern MW. 1993. EpiMAN: a spatial decision support system for use in an exotic disease emergency. *Agricultural Systems and Information Technology* **5**: 20-22.

Sanson RL, Morris RS, Stern MW. 1997. The epidemiological management system (EpiMan). Proceedings, Epidemiology Program, 10th FAVA Congress, Cairns Australia. pp 171-176.

Sanson RL, Pfeiffer DU. Morris RS. 1994. Geographic information systems: their application in animal disease control. *Rev. Sci. Tech. Off. Int. Epi.* **10**: 179-195.

Scott-Orr H. 1985. *Surveillance for bovine tuberculosis: the efficiency of an abattoir traceback system.* Proceedings of the 4th International Symposium on Veterinary Epidemiology and economics 18-22 November 1985, Singapore pp 374-376.

Scudamore JM. 1988. Disease reporting systems in Great Britain. *Revue Scientifique et Technical d'Office International des Epizooties* **7**

Sergeant ESG, Cameron AR, Baldock FC, Vongthilath S. 1997. An animal health information system for Laos. Proceedings, Epidemiology Program, 10th FAVA Congress, Cairns Australia. pp 157-160.

Sharma P. 1994. Use of geographic information systems in animal health information programs. In: Copland JW, Gleeson LJ, Chamnanpood C. (eds) *Diagnosis and epidemiology of foot-and-mouth disease in Southeast Asia. Proceedings of an international workshop held at Lampang, Thailand, September 6-9, 1993*, Vol. ACIAR Proceedings No. 51. Australian Centre for International Agricultural Research, Canberra. pp 119-125.

Sharma VP, Srivastava A. 1997. Role of geographic information system in malaria control. *Indian Journal Medical Research* **106**: 198-204.

Shaw J. 1992. Sentinel herd study of bluetongue virus in Puerto Rico. Preliminary results, January 1991. *Annals New York Academy of Science* **653**: 194-196

Smith, G.S., (1989) Development of rapid epidemiologic assessment methods to evaluate health status and delivery of health services. *International Journal of Epidemiology* **18**:S2-S15

Stärk KDC. 1996. Animal health monitoring and surveillance in Switzerland. *Australian Veterinary Journal* **73**:96-97

Stärk, KDC, Frei PP, Frei-Stoheli C. 1994. The health profile of Swiss dairy cows - a contribution to integrated animal health information. *The Kenya Veterinarian* **18**:48-50

Stärk KDC, Vicari A, Kihm U, Nicolet J. 1995. Surveillance of contagious bovine pleuropneumonia in Switzerland. *Rev. sci. tech. Off. Int. Epiz.* **14:** 621- 629.

St George TD. 1980. A sentinel herd system for the study of arbovirus infections in Australia and Papua New Guinea. *Veterinary Science Communications* **4**: 39-51.

St George TD. 1985. Studies on the pathogenesis of bovine ephemeral fever in sentinel cattle. I. Virology and serology. *Veterinary Microbiology* **10**: 493-504.

Thai Department of Livestock Development. 1994. *1994 Annual Reprot of the Livestock Development Office Region 5.* Department of Livestock Development, Thailand.

Thieme A. 1983. Modelling the cost and benefits of foot and mouth disease control programs. Proceedings 3rd International Symposium on Veterinary Epidemiology and Economics pp 384-391.

Thrusfield M. 1995. Sources of data. In: Veterinary epidemiology, second edition. Blackwell Science, Oxford. pp 143-150.

Touray, G.M. (1990) A plan for PARC rinderpest seriological surveillance in the Gambia. In: *The sero-monitoring of rinderpest throughout Africa. Phase One. Proceedings of a Final Research Co-ordination*

Meeting of the FAO/IAEA/SIDA/OAU/IBAR/PARC Coordinated Research Programme, Bingerville, Cote d'Ivoire, 19-23 November, 1990. International Atomic Energy Agency (IAEA), Vienna, pp 145-147.

Tounkara, K., Diallo, B.O., Sangare, K.O., Seck, B. and Traore, A. (1990) Report on the sero-monitoring programme in Mali. In: *The sero-monitoring of rinderpest throughout Africa. Phase One. Proceedings of a Final Research Co-ordination Meeting of the FAO/IAEA/SIDA/OAU/IBAR/PARC Coordinated Research Programme, Bingerville, Cote d'Ivoire, 19-23 November, 1990.* International Atomic Energy Agency (IAEA), Vienna, pp 167-178.

Turner AG, Magnani RJ, Shuaib M. 1996. A not quite as quick but much cleaner alternative to the expanded programme on immunization (EPI) cluster survey design. *International Journal of Epidemiology* **25**:198-203

Tyler L. 1990. PARC sero-monitoring: Survey design, implementation and the analysis, presentation and use of results. In: *The sero-monitoring of rinderpest throughout Africa. Phase One. Proceedings of a Final Research Co-ordination Meeting of the FAO/IAEA/SIDA/OAU/IBAR/PARC Coordinated Research Programme, Bingerville, Cote d'Ivoire, 19-23 November, 1990.* International Atomic Energy Agency (IAEA), Vienna, 67-80

United States Animals Health Association (1987) Automation of animal health programs. In: *Proceedings of 91st Annual Meeting of the United States Animal Health Association, Salt Lake City, Utah, October 25-30, 1987.* United States Animal Health Association, Richmond, pp 114-123.

Van der Logt PB, Morris RS, Hathaway SC. 1994.The analysis of chemical residue data gathered at abattoirs by means of geographical information systems. *The Kenya Veterinarian* **18**:496-498

Vongthilath S. in press. Country Report - Lao PDR. In: Sharma P. (ed) *Proceedings of the International Workshop on a Regional Computerised Animal Health Information System, June 3-5, 1997, Vientiane, Lao PDR.* Australian Centre for International Agricultural Research, Canberra.
Sollod AE, Stem C. 1991. Appropriate animal health information systems for nomadic and transhumant livestock population in Africa. *Revue Scientifique et Technical d'Office International des Epizooties* **10**:89-101

Vonk Noordegraaf A, Buijtels JA, Dijkhuizen AA, Franken P, Stegeman JA, Verhoeff J. 1998. An epidemiological and economic simulation model to evaluate the spread and control of infectious bovine rhinotracheitis in The Netherlands. *Preventive Veterinary Medicine* **36**(3):219-38

Waltner-Toews D, Bernardo TM, Stemshorn BW. 1991. The Caribbean animal and plant health information network (CARAPHIN) : Animal Health. In: Martin, S.W. (ed) *Proceedings of the 6th ISVEE symposium, Ottawa, Canada, 12-16 August, 1991.* University of Guelph, Ontario, pp 645-645.

Ward MP, Flanagan M, Carpenter TE, Hird DW, Thurmond MC, Johnson SJ, Dashorst ME. 1995. Infection of cattle with bluetongue viruses in Queensland, Australia: results of a sentinel herd study, 1990-1992. *Veterinary Microbiology* **45**: 35-44.

Washino RK, Wood BL. 1994. Application of remote sensing to arthropod vector surveillance and control. *American Journal Tropical Medicine and Hygiene* **50**(6 Suppl): 134-144.

Wilesmith JW, Wells GA, Cranwell MP, Ryan JB. 1988. Bovine spongioform encephalopathy: epidemiological studies. *Veterinary Record* **123**: 638-644.

Willeberg P. (1985) Epidemiologic use of routinely collected veterinary data: risks and benefits. In: *Proceedings of the 4th International Symposium on Veterinary Epidemiology & Economics, Singapore, 18-22 November, 1985.* International Society for Veterinary Epidemiology and Economics (ISVEE), Singapore, 40-45

Wilson GWC. 1987. The foot and mouth disease epidemic 1967/68. *State Veterinary Journal* **119**: 97-102

Yip PSF, Bruno G, Tajima N, Seber GAF, Buckland ST, Cormack RM, Unwin N, Chang Y-F, Fienberg SE, Junker BW, LaPorte RE, Libman IM, McCarty DJ. (1995) Capture-recapture and multiple record systems estimation II: Applications in human diseases. *American Journal of Epidemiology* **142**:1059-1068

Chapter 3

Advances in Diagnostic Technology

3.1 Introduction

The objective of this chapter is to describe the development of current diagnostic technology and its application to livestock diseases. It should enable the reader to understand the benefits of new technologies over older methods, how certain technologies are applied and to anticipate future developments. Examples are drawn from the major transboundary animal diseases as appropriate.

As our knowledge has improved of the structure and function of pathogens and of the immunological responses of a host to infection or antigenic stimulation, approaches to both disease diagnosis and to immunisation have changed from empirical methodologies to procedures undertaken in a much more informed manner. These approaches have enabled diagnostic assays to become more specific and better standardised and have resulted in the development of vaccines of greater safety and efficacy and of a more reliable quality. Advances in laboratory technology have enabled diagnostic assays to be performed and anlaysed with a greater degree of automation, with improved precision and reduced labour requirements. However, some of these advances come at an increased cost and it is therefore not always appropriate to apply them, especially with the strong budgetary constraints of most developing countries. We now have the scientific knowledge and technical skills available to make very significant further advances in the diagnosis of, and immunisation against, specific diseases. Such expected advances will also be highlighted in the following discussion.

3.2 Overview

Laboratory diagnostic technology is directed toward either:

(a) detection of the presence or absence of a pathogen and its subsequent identification and characterisation; or
(b) detection of the pathological effect of, or immunological response to, infection by a particular pathogen.

In the past, detection of a pathogen has been achieved by visualisation of the organism by light or electron microscopy, either directly in specimens from the affected animal or after culture. Alternatively, serological procedures are used in which specific antigen is detected using known antisera. There have been significant advances made in such serological procedures, the most important of which will be described in following Sections.

Polymerase chain replication (PCR) technology represents an entirely new technology and this is described in Section 3.9. *In vitro* bacterial or viral culture is widely used to isolate and multiply a pathogen, so that the organism itself, or its antigen, can be more readily detected, by virtue of being present in greater quantity and generally with fewer contaminants. PCR technology permits the same principle (ie, *in vitro* amplification) to be applied to the detection of specific sequences of nucleic acid. There are enormous benefits to this approach, but it is currently limited by deficiencies in knowledge and by cost. It can be expected that these limitations will be progressively (and probably rapidly) addressed and that this technology will be applied to an increasing extent in the future.

There have been enormous advances in our understanding of immunology. However, with a few exceptions, immunological approaches to infectious disease diagnosis are directed toward serological procedures – ie, the detection of interactions between antigens unique to the pathogen and specific antibodies elaborated against them. Serological procedures are applied to detection and characterisation of a pathogen, as described above. However, they are applied in greater volume to detecting and measuring antibody responses and this is the emphasis given in the following sections.

The most important advance in laboratory technology has been in the development of microtitration techniques (Section 3.3) and in particular, its application to enzyme immunoassay (Section 3.4). Together, these technologies have permitted serological procedures to be undertaken more cost-effectively and with better standardisation. They have also facilitated direct downloading of data to computers for recording, analysis and transmission of results. This has not only reduced labour and the potential for errors, but has improved inter-laboratory and international standardisation and collaboration in diagnostic testing and its application to disease control.

3.3 Laboratory methodologies

Serological assays were originally carried out in test tubes. Relatively large volumes of reagents were required and assays involving large numbers of tubes were cumbersome. Glassware required careful washing before re-use, to remove all of the assay products and reagents and to avoid cross-contamination. Virus neutralisation tests were commonly undertaken in glass flasks or petri dishes.

Over time, disposable plastic has largely replaced glass, greatly improving the reliability of assays because of the difficulty of achieving adequate cleanliness of washed glassware. This has come at a cost, which is generally acceptable in developed countries where it is offset by greater savings in the labour required for washing. In developing countries where labour costs are generally lower and plasticware is commonly imported and therefore requires foreign exchange, cost it is still a constraint in moving from glass to plasticware.

Attempts were made for many years to reduce reagent volumes in serological assays. Some agglutination tests, using a stained antigen for ease of visualising a reaction, were readily adapted to small volumes by placing reagents as drops onto microscope slides. Haemagglutination assays were carried out in wells in perspex 'WHO' plates in volumes of less than 1 ml. A virus neutralisation (VN) assay for antibody to foot and mouth disease (FMD) virus was developed in moulded plastic plates, with the assay being read by eye on the basis of a pH-related colour change.

In the 1960s, serological assays using 96-well microplates were developed, with reactant volumes of 25µl or 50 µl and a total assay volume of 50µl to 250 µl. This has now become the standard format for conducting a wide range of assays. Plates of essentially the same dimensions are manufactured by a large number of suppliers. Wells of different shapes (V, U or flat based) are used for different assays. Plastics of different composition, or treated in a variety of ways after manufacture, are used for particular applications.

Together with microplates, a large range of equipment has been developed to dispense reagents, incubate plates (often with shaking), wash plates and read reactions, usually by spectrophotometry. Microplate readers generally can be interfaced with a computer and/or have a microprocessor and software to enable data to be processed, analysed and printed.

While microplate technology has been universally adopted in the developed world, there are still some issues that need to be considered in applying it in developing countries. Microtitration plates and pipetting tips are generally regarded as disposable but they do represent a significant cost. Sometimes this plasticware can be washed and re-used several times. Microtitration plates can often be re-used for assays such as agglutination or HAI, which are not dependent on particular properties of the plastic surface. Pipette tips can more commonly be re-used, provided they are well washed using a non-ionic detergent, well rinsed and, where appropriate, adequately sterilised. When plasticware is re-used, additional quality control procedures should be considered to ensure that inadequate washing does not contribute to variation between tests.

For VN assays, microplates are usually (but not always) required that have been treated to ensure that cell culture monolayers will form and have been gamma irradiated and appropriately packaged to ensure that they are sterile. For certain ELISAs, particular plates that will optimise adsorption of immunoreactants and/or minimise adsorption of interfering contaminants are often required. Sometimes the development of a particular assay has involved a comparison of microplates to find the most suitable one for an application. Careful comparative studies, together with advice from international laboratories will generally indicate which assays must be carried out with particular microplates and which ones can have plates substituted. While lower cost is usually the reason for the latter decision, there can be general benefits in a laboratory for one type of microplate to be used for a number of applications.

It is likely that the future will provide attractive alternatives to microtitration technology. Disposable testing kits that can be used almost anywhere with a minimum of technical expertise will become more widely available. However, the complex manufacturing technology required will dictate that they are produced commercially and their availability will be limited, especially for application to transboundary diseases of livestock, by the quantitative demand for tests and the ability of prospective users to pay for them.

Microtitration technology does not lend itself to process automation. It can be expected that immunoassay techniques will be developed for the kind of automatic analysers that are currently used in clinical laboratories for biochemical and endocrinological assays. Again, such developments are probably many years away for widespread veterinary application and are unlikely to be a good prospect for developing countries in which labour costs are not the major constraint. In conclusion, microplate technology is likely to continue as the appropriate technology for immunoassay for livestock diseases in the foreseeable future.

3.4 Enzyme immunoassay

3.4.1 Techniques

Immunological assay procedures depend on the detection of an interaction between antigen and antibody. In the past, assays were developed around properties of antibodies, which enabled detection to take place. Some formed complexes with antigen, which were large enough to be detectable by eye and were visualised as agglutination reactions (where clumped complexes are seen in suspension) or immunodiffusion reactions (where precipitation is seen at the interface of antigen and antibody diffusing toward each other in a gel). Others fixed complement, which was then unavailable to lyse sensitised erythrocytes. Others neutralised infectious virus, which then failed to grow in tissue culture to produce a visible cytopathic effect.

Over time, methods were developed to detect antigen/antibody reactions, which could not be otherwise visualised. Fluorescent compounds were attached to either antigen or antibody so that interactions could be detected by examination under ultraviolet light. Radioisotopes were used as a marker, with a reaction detected by counting the emissions of β- or γ-particles by appropriate procedures.

All of these procedures had certain particular disadvantages that limited their application. Agglutination tests are generally not very sensitive, because large concentrations of reactants are required to see the reaction by the naked eye. Also it is difficult to express reactions in an accurate and quantitative manner – often they are expressed as negative or positive (+ to ++++). Complement fixation tests can be quantified accurately and even automated. But they are subject to variation because of the large number of biological reagents involved (complement, haemolysin, erythrocytes) which can vary over time and/or with different sources. Neutralisation tests require the use of live infectious organisms, requiring careful control of culture conditions to achieve the correct infectivity titre and to avoid contamination and, occasionally, to protect workers from infection. Immunofluorescent and radioisotope procedures generally require expensive equipment and, in the case of radioisotopes, represent a potential health risk to workers.

Ultimately, a solution was developed to detecting a serological reaction (ie, a reaction between antigen and antibody), by a method which could be applied widely and which suffered from few of the disadvantages of other procedures. This was achieved by attaching an enzyme to one of the immunoreactants, which could be detected at very low concentration by reacting it with a substrate to produce a coloured product. This can be seen by eye or measured for concentration by a spectrophotometer. Appropriate control reactions must also be included to provide known negative and positive results.

The principle of enzyme immunoassay can be summarised as follows:

- Specific antigen and antibody are allowed to react. For antibody measurement, known antigen is reacted with unknown sample, which may contain specific antibody. For antigen detection, a known antiserum is used.
- An enzyme is introduced into the system. This may either be conjugated to the known specific reagent (usually antibody) or else be added in an additional step. An enzyme is used which, when reacted with a particular substrate, results in the production of a coloured product.
- Immunoreagents that have bound to each other are separated from unreacted reagents.
- Substrate is added.
- The extent of binding between antigen and antibody is determined by the development of a coloured product.

The most popular application of the technology is enzyme-linked immunosorbent assay (ELISA), in which reactants are progressively bound to a solid surface (commonly a microplate). Separation can then be achieved by washing unbound reactant away from that bound to the surface, before proceeding with addition of the next reagent. Enzyme immunoassay can also be applied to detecting antigen in tissue sections or smears. However, immunofluorescence is often still preferred to immunoperoxidase procedures and there are few instances where these procedures are applied to the major transboundary diseases. The following discussion is therefore directed specifically to ELISA. There are many good overviews of immunoassay, one being Price and Newman (1997).

A large number of different ELISA procedures have been developed. In a *direct ELISA*, antigen is detected with enzyme conjugated specific antibody. In an *indirect ELISA*, the specific antigen and antibody is reacted and then detected with a third, enzyme-conjugated anti-species antibody. This has the benefit of enabling one enzyme-conjugated anti-species reagent to be used for assays for a range of pathogens. The additional step also results in an amplification of the signal, as more enzyme is bound. In a *sandwich ELISA*, antigen is trapped by one antibody and detected with another. Antigen detection ELISAs are generally of this kind because the initial solid phase coating step is non-specific and it is not appropriate to apply an unknown specimen in this way. Some other variations of ELISA are described in the examples given below but these are not comprehensive. Among the alternatives to ELISA is dot immunobinding, in which the solid phase is a nitrocellulose or nylon membrane and very small volumes of specimens are applied as multiple spots, usually for a qualitative assessment as a positive or negative result (Towbin and Gordon, 1984; Singh and Singh, 1997).

ELISA is a form of heterogeneous immunoassay, in which bound label is separated from free label by washing steps. The performance of such assays is dependent on the specificity of binding and efficient separation of bound and unbound label. Homogeneous assays on the other hand, depend on modulation of the signal of the label when antigen is bound to antibody compared to when it is free. Avoidance of a separation step can greatly simplify the procedure, which can be particularly important for automation and for field or pen-side kit systems (for example, see Section 3.6.2.4).

Other variations of heterogeneous immunoassay are those utilising chemiluminescence or fluorescence, both of which are potentially more sensitive that ELISA. However, in practice, exquisite sensitivity is not generally required for infectious disease diagnosis and the benefits of these alternative procedures would not justify the investment in an alternative technology.

There are a number of very important benefits of ELISA, which have made it the most commonly applied serological assay system in use today. Equipment and consumables are readily available from many sources. Universal reagents such as enzyme and substrate can be purchased commercially, are safe and can be stored for long periods. Anti-species conjugates are available for detecting antibody to most livestock and laboratory animal species. As ELISA diagnostic procedures for particular diseases become widely adopted, specific antigen and/or antisera are often available from international reference sources and sometimes kits are available containing all consumables for an assay.

Because the technology can be applied to a wide range of disease diagnostic procedures, it is usually advantageous for a laboratory to standardise on ELISA, rather than having to maintain resources and staff skills for several alternative procedures. The ability to read assays on a microplate spectrophotometer and download results a computer for analysis, further manipulation or transmission to others, is often the stimulus for changing from older methodologies to ELISA.

However, there are some important considerations for successfully applying ELISA technology. Appropriate equipment should be selected, taking into account test volume and budgetary constraints. For many laboratories, an ELISA might involve no more than two to four microplates. In this situation, reagents are best added with single- or multi-channel micropipettes. Washing is readily achieved with a squeeze bottle and small, purpose-built shaker-incubators are available, specifically for application to ELISA. Microplate readers vary in cost and sophistication. Some tests can be read by eye. Most require a reader, with the appropriate filter for measurement of optical density at a particular wavelength. If ELISA technology is to be widely applied in a laboratory, it is usually advisable to have a reader which can be used for a number of different wavelengths (for different substrates) and which can be interfaced with a computer for data analysis.

Attention to detail is essential for accurate and repeatable results. If any change is to be made in reagents or test conditions, thorough comparative studies must be conducted to ensure that results are the same or vary in a predictable manner. Appropriate controls are necessary to monitor background, non-specific reactions and specific reactions with positive samples at known concentrations. While there are benefits for a laboratory in standardising microplates, buffers, conjugates and substrates for a variety of applications, assays prescribed for international trade (OIE, 1996) should not be modified without the agreement of all interested parties, including affected trading partners.

ELISA results must be interpreted with care. Generally, the range of optical densities obtained with true positive samples will overlap with the range for true negative samples. Cut-off limits must be defined. In different circumstances, it may be necessary to ensure that no positive reactions are missed (so the cut-off is set low) or that no negative results are missed (so the cut-off is set high) – ie the sensitivity and specificity are somewhat interdependent – see Section 1.4. Occasionally a range in indeterminate results is defined, between the positive and negative cut-off limits.

3.4.2 Applications

In this and following Sections (3.4, 3.5 and 3.7), examples are given of the application of ELISA to the major transboundary diseases. The emphasis is on describing the different assay procedures from the point of view of the principles involved and they should not be followed as laboratory procedures. The OIE Manual of Standards for Diagnostic Techniques and Vaccines (OIE, 1996) is the key resource for determining which assays are currently applied to particular infectious diseases.

3.4.2.1 FMD antigen ELISA

This assay enables detection of FMD viral antigen to any of the seven types (O, A, C, SAT1, SAT2, SAT3, Asia1). (Roeder and Le Blanc Smith, 1987; Ferris and Dawson, 1988). Because the major (146s) antigen involved is type specific, the procedure involves performing a separate assay for each antigen. In endemically infected countries, it is common to test only for those types which are expected.

Prior to the use of ELISA, FMD antigen detection was undertaken by complement fixation test (CFT), either in tubes or in microplates. This was a reliable procedure and under optimum conditions is of comparable sensitivity to ELISA. Apart from occasional samples producing anti-complementary results by CFT, the main reason for better results being obtained by current ELISA procedures is that antiserum production methods have been improved to ensure that the predominant antibody is to 146s antigen and has broad intratypic reactivity (Ferris, 1988).

The assay can be used for detecting FMD viral antigen in specimens collected from an animal (in particular, vesicular epithelium) or in culture fluids from tissue culture cell monolayers inoculated with a specimen. It provides a rapid determination of the presence of FMD viral antigen and simultaneously identifies the virus type.

The steps involved in the assay are described below. Between each step, plates are incubated and washed. Appropriate control wells are included.

1. To separate rows, rabbit antiserum to each particular virus type is added.
2. Samples of the unknown specimen are added to wells in each row, in a range a dilutions.
3. Guinea pig antiserum for each particular virus type is added at a pre-determined dilution to the appropriate row.
4. Rabbit anti-guinea pig serum, conjugated to enzyme (horseradish peroxidase) is added to each well.
5. Substrate (orthophenylene diamine) is added to each well.

Colour development will occur in wells in which FMD viral antigen of a particular type has bound the type-specific rabbit immunoglobulin. In turn, the type specific guinea pig antibody is bound to the viral antigen, the rabbit serum-enzyme conjugate is bound to the guinea pig immunoglobulin and the substrate-enzyme reaction occurs in wells in which the enzyme conjugate is present. Specificity of the assay is enhanced by the fact that both the capture (guinea pig) antiserum and the detection (rabbit) antiserum are FMD virus type-specific.

Cross-reactions between virus types can occur but are generally at a lower level than the specific type reaction. It should be borne in mind that on rare occasions animals can be concurrently infected with more than one FMD virus type and antigen of both types may be detected in the same specimen (Woodbury *et al.*, 1994).

3.4.2.2 FMD antibody ELISA

Prior to the introduction of ELISA for FMD antibody measurement, virus neutralisation tests were used. For diagnostic application including epidemiological and vaccine efficacy studies, these had been adapted to a microtitration format. Virus neutralisation tests are notoriously difficult to control due to the large number of factors that can affect cell metabolism and virus production. Tests must be performed under sterile conditions and they also represent a potential hazard for spread of infection, since infectious virus must be used. Furthermore, the assay takes several days before a result is available. These factors have often limited their application to countries in which FMD (and the particular virus type) is endemic and/or to laboratories with appropriate microbiological containment.

However, protection against FMD is closely correlated to neutralising antibody levels and so the titres of antibody measured in virus neutralisation tests is a good predictor of protection or indicator of vaccine efficacy. Consequently, when an ELISA was developed to replace the VN test, it was important that it should also detect neutralising antibody. A procedure was developed in which the reaction between antigen and antibody occurs in liquid phase – the liquid-phase blocking ELISA (OIE, 1996). If desired for microbiological security, antigens can be inactivated prior to use.

In the first (liquid-phase) part of the assay, antigen of a particular FMD virus type and at a pre-determined concentration is incubated with the serum sample at a range of dilutions. This is carried out in a carrier plate (not an ELISA plate). The reaction between the antigen and any antibody present in the sample takes place in the liquid medium and is comparable to a virus neutralisation reaction. Samples from each well are then transferred to an ELISA plate and unbound antigen is assayed in a system identical to the FMD antigen ELISA described above. In wells in which specific antibody is present in the serum sample, FMD antigen is bound and there is a diminished level of antigen detected in the ELISA.

3.4.2.3 ELISA for antibody to Rift Valley fever virus

An indirect ELISA was developed, using inactivated antigen, purified from cell culture monolayers such that it could be used for direct coating of microplates (Paweska *et al.*, 1995). Antibody in serum samples was captured by the antigen and detected using enzyme-conjugated protein G. Protein G binds to immunoglobulin molecules, including IgM, of many animal species, so that this assay can be applied to detect recent infection in a range of animals, without the need for separate antispecies conjugates. The ELISA correlated 100% with HI and compared to the virus neutralisation test, had a sensitivity and specificity both of >97%.

3.5 Specificity of serological assays

The terms *sensitivity* and *specificity* are applied to tests used to determine the presence of a disease, or antibody to a pathogen, in an animal populations. The *sensitivity* of a test is the percentage of true positive specimens that will have a positive result. If a test is 100% sensitive, there are no false-negative results. The *specificity* of a test is the percentage of true negative specimens that will have a negative result. A test that is 100% specific will produce no false-positive results. In practice, no serological assay can be expected to be either 100% sensitive or 100% specific and this needs to be taken into account when evaluating the results of tests (see Chapter 2).

The sensitivity of a test is dependent on the kind of assay that is used and the conditions under which it is applied. It is also dependent on the specific immunoreactants that are used. For example, a broadly reactive antiserum that is used for antigen detection is more likely to detect a pathogen across the full range of its antigenic spectrum. The specificity of a test is dependent on these factors, often in a reciprocal manner. Thus, an antiserum which is too broadly reactive may in fact have a high sensitivity but low specificity, because it also detects antigen to distantly related viruses that are not of concern. This reactivity of antibodies is also referred to as *specificity*, being the ability of an antibody to distinguish a particular target structure (antigenic site, or epitope) from other structures from which we wish to differentiate the target. Similarly, antigens used to detect antibodies to a particular pathogen can vary in their ability to specifically bind only to the target antibodies.

Much of the research and development involved in the development of a new procedure is directed toward finding assay conditions and immunoreagents that will optimise the *efficiency* of a test. This is the percentage of all test results, positive or negative, that are correct. Achieving the greatest efficiency will usually require some compromise between optimum sensitivity and optimum specificity.

Two advances in molecular biology have given us greatly improved opportunities to improve the specific reactivity of immunoreagents. The development of hybridoma technology has enabled us to produce and select monoclonal antibodies (MAbs) with the particular reactivity that is sought. The production of isolated antigenic components *in vitro* by recombinant DNA techniques or even by *de novo* synthesis from constituent amino acids has provided a similar potential for antigen of highly defined reactivity. With such reagents capable of producing results of high *specificity*, assay development with them can then be focussed on achieving optimum *sensitivity*. The immediate benefit is a test of greater efficiency. However, these approaches also present the opportunity for producing essentially unlimited, uniformly reactive batches of reagents, which can be widely distributed and greatly facilitate the standardisation of testing within and between laboratories.

3.6 Monoclonal antibodies

3.6.1 Techniques

Polyclonal antiserum to a particular pathogen can vary in specificity and affinity according to the immunising antigen and the immunising regime, the use or otherwise of adjuvants, the time of bleeding an immunised animal and other variable factors. With exactly the same immunisation procedure, different animals may respond differently, both quantitatively and qualitatively, in respect of the antibody produced. Thus, different batches of an antiserum will almost certainly perform differently, to a greater or lesser extent, when used in a serological procedure.

An animal responds to immunisation by producing antibodies of varying specificity and affinity and directed toward different epitopes, because they are elaborated by cells originating from different stem cells. Monoclonal antibodies (MAbs) are produced by hybrid cells. The parent cell is produced by fusing a competent antibody-producing cell with a cell possessing the properties required for *in vitro* replication. The principle steps in MAb production are:

1. Mice are immunised with the antigen of interest, to stimulate the development of clones of antibody-producing cells from pre-existing stem cells.
2. The mice are killed, spleen cells removed and mixed with mouse myeloma cells in the presence of polyethylene glycol to obtain fusion between the two cell types. A special culture medium is used in which only hybrid cells will grow (HAT medium).
3. Hybrid cells resulting from the fusion are grown in microplates.
4. Colonies are assayed for antibody production. It is important that the assay be simple and specific, as a large number of colonies may need to be screened. Also, the assay should be consistent with the intended use of the MAb – for example, a MAb that reacts with an antigen in solution, may not do so when it is bound to a surface in an ELISA. Other properties of the MAb may subsequently need to be determined, such as its affinity and its immunoglobulin class.

5. Candidate colonies are cloned three times by limiting dilution to ensure that the resulting culture is the progeny of one cell only and that the product is therefore a monoclonal antibody.
6. Positive cultures are passaged and cells frozen for long-term storage
7. Large quantities of MAbs are produced most commonly by generating tumors in mice with the hybridoma cells and harvesting the antibody-rich ascitic fluid. However, *in vitro* methods for large-scale culture of hybridoma cells are becoming more widely used and will ultimately replace ascites production. In any event, harvests generally undergo some degree of purification, often by affinity chromatography, in which MAb is bound by antigen or by protein A and subsequently eluted.

Once a hybridoma cell line is established, it can be passaged in cell culture and stored frozen. Production of the MAb is therefore 'immortalised' and it will always be of the same reactivity. This is the most important property of MAbs as diagnostic reagents, since they can be distributed widely and used over a long period of time to obtain comparable results.

There are alternative procedures to hybridoma technology for producing MAbs, which are under development but unlikely to be applied to diagnostic technology for some years to come. These include the production of transgenic mice carrying a particular immunoglobulin gene from a different species, the reconstruction of MAbs by genetic engineering to direct them toward a particular application, the introduction of immunoglobulin genes into bacterial expression systems to produce the specific variable fragments of an antibody and the expression of complete antibody genes in mammalian cells (Zola, 1995).

Despite the benefits of MAbs, there are drawbacks to their use as diagnostic reagents. Their specificity dictates that they must be directed to highly conserved epitopes. Such epitopes may not have the antigenic properties that distinguish the target pathogen from unrelated organisms. They may not be present in large numbers and the affinity of the binding between the antibody and the epitope may not be high. Polyclonal antisera, because they contain antibodies directed toward a range of epitopes on different parts of the target molecule, will often have the broader reactivity required to ensure that all variants of the pathogen are detected. Polyclonal antisera also bind both more strongly and form larger antigen-antibody aggregates, which can be important for assays involving precipitation, such as agglutination tests. For ELISAs, which do not depend on precipitation, one solution is to employ mixtures of MAbs to obtain the required spread of reactivity. To a large extent, the limitation of lower binding of MAbs can be compensated by the fact that high quality anti-mouse conjugates can be obtained commercially, so that detection of bound MAb is generally efficient.

3.6.2 Applications

3.6.2.1 Rinderpest antibody ELISA

This is a competitive ELISA, in which rinderpest antibody in a specimen is detected and measured by its ability to compete with a MAb for binding to rinderpest viral antigen (OIE, 1996). The MAb (designated as C1) reacts with the haemagglutinin protein of rinderpest virus. Microplates are incubated and washed after each step and appropriate controls are included.

1. Wells of a microplate are coated with rinderpest antigen.
2. Test serum samples, immediately followed by MAb, are added to the wells.
3. Enzyme-conjugated rabbit anti-mouse immunglobulin is added to the wells.
4. Substrate is added.

The presence of specific antibody in a sample reduces binding of the MAb and subsequently results in a reduced development of colour.

This assay has been applied to samples collected as dried whole blood on filter paper (Heller *et al.*, 1998). This requires the collection of only very small amounts of sample and transport to a testing laboratory are facilitated without the need for samples to be kept cold. Compared to the use of conventionally prepared serum samples, testing was 100% sensitive and more than 98% specific.

3.6.2.2 ELISA for CBPP serology

A monoclonal antibody, designated 117/5, reacted with 183 strains of *Mycoplasma mycoides* subsp. *mycoides* SC (the aetiological agent of contagious bovine pleuropneumonia – CBPP) but not with any other *Mycoplasma* species (Le Goff *et al.*, 1998). The ELISA involved coating plates with antigen prepared washed organisms lysed with detergent. Serum samples for testing were diluted and mixed with monoclonal antibody in a strict competitive assay. When compared with the CFT, the ELISA was 96% sensitive and 97% specific. In selecting a cutoff, sensitivity was sacrificed in the interests of specificity. However, comparison with the CFT, with which false positive reactions have been identified and antibody is only detectable for an average of 30 days after infection, may not give a good indication of the true specificity. This assay is currently undergoing final field evaluation before being adopted as the serological test of choice for CBPP. Current information (January, 1999) is that on the basis of more extensive field trials, the assay is ≥99% specific and at least as sensitive at the CFT, in detecting infection. It will however, not detect antibody resulting from vaccination (R.Geiger, pers. comm.).

3.6.2.3 Differentiation between rinderpest and PPR viruses

Rinderpest and PPR can both affect small ruminants, may cause similar clinical signs and may both be present in the same geographic area. Experimental animal inoculation or virus isolation and identification are time-consuming approaches to differentiating the viruses. An immunocapture ELISA can be used to rapidly differentiate rinderpest and PPR viral antigens in clinical specimens (Libeau *et al.*, 1994). In this assay, binding of enzyme is achieved through a reaction between biotin and streptavidin. Antibodies are readily labelled with biotin and enzymes with avidin and the reaction between biotin and avidin is essential irreversible (Kendal *et al.*, 1983). Microplates are incubated and washed after each step and appropriate controls are included.

1. Microplates are coated with a MAb that reacts with the nucleoprotein of both viruses.
2. Sample suspension is added to the wells
3. Biotinylated MAbs specific for epitopes on the nucleoprotein of either rinderpest virus or PPR virus are added to separate wells and streptavidin-peroxidase is added to all wells.
4. Substrate is added.

A colour develops in the wells in which the biotinylated Mab corresponds to the viral antigen that is present.

3.6.2.4 A pen-side test for rinderpest viral antigen

This is one of the few immunoassays that have been developed for livestock disease diagnosis in the field. In can detect antigen in ocular discharges of affected animals and can be performed in five minutes.

The system is patented and will be commercially marketed. Antigen in a specimen is bound to dyed, MAb-labelled microspheres which migrate along a nitrocellulose membrane (IAH, 1994). The complex is bound by an immobilised band of trapping antibody, resulting in the development of a coloured band. A control band of anti-mouse antibody further along the strip confirms that the MAb has migrated past the anti-rinderpest trapping antibody. The test is rinderpest-specific and has a similar sensitivity to the immunocapture ELISA described in Section 3.6 above. (IAH, 1995)

3.6.2.5 Antigenic comparison of FMD virus isolates

The most important application of antigenic analysis of FMD virus isolates is to monitor the ability of vaccine strains in use to protect against currently circulating field strains. The virus neutralisation reaction is the most appropriate *in vivo* reference system as it involves the antigenic determinants responsible for protective immunity (Rweyemamu, 1984). The liquid-phase blocking ELISA (see Section 1.3.2) produces comparable results. However, it is possible to more readily detect small antigenic differences using MAbs and these can be selected so that they are reactive with the known epitopes of the virus that are responsible for neutralisation. A variety of approaches have been used. Davidson *et al.* (1995) used a sandwich ELISA and developed MAb-binding profiles, which were compared by hierarchical cluster analysis.

3.7 Recombinant antigens

Nucleic acid technology has revolutionised infectious disease diagnosis. It has introduced the era in which nucleic acid detection can be used as a means of identifying the presence of a pathogen in a clinical specimen and this is discussed in Section 3.9.

It has also provided a means by which highly purified and characterised antigens can be prepared and utilised in serological assays. Such antigens can provide, in common with MAbs, a source of reagent that is essentially unlimited and with known and constant properties, with substantial benefits for standardisation and for providing reagents to laboratories that do not have their own facilities for reagent preparation. The principles of the technology are outlined in Chapter 4

3.7.1 Application

3.7.1.1 PPR antibody ELISA

The prescribed test for PPR serology is a VN test (OIE, 1996). Cross-reactions occur in this procedure between antibody to rinderpest virus and PPR antibody. Consequently to discriminate antibodies to the two viruses, cross-neutralisation tests may be required, using both viruses, with the higher neutralisation titre being taken to represent the specific response. A competitive ELISA has been developed, which is the same in principle as that described for rinderpest in 1.5.1 above. However, this test is specific for PPR antibody by virtue of employing a recombinant PPR nucleoprotein produced in a baculovirus (Libeau *et al.*, 1995).

3.8 Immunoblotting

3.8.1 Techniques

Polypeptides of denatured proteins can be separated according to their molecular size and electrical charge by migration through a gel matrix in an electrical field. The greater the charge of a molecule, or the smaller its size, the more rapidly it will migrate through the gel towards an oppositely charged electrode. Typically, separation is carried out in a polyacrylamide or agarose-acrylamide gel. Proteins are denatured with sodium dodecyl sulphate (SDS), which confers a net negative charge and migration occurs toward the cathode at a rate, which is proportional to the molecular mass of the protein.

Separated polypeptides can be compared with proteins of a known molecular mass, run in parallel, to determine their molecular masses. Denatured proteins from different sources (for example, from different isolates of a virus) can also be compared by running them in parallel lanes of a gel. Differentiation of polypeptides on the basis of their isoelectric point (electrofocusing) can be achieved by running the denatured proteins in a pH gradient such that they migrate to a pH at which their net charge is zero. This technique has been used to compare strains of FMD virus isolated from the field or used in vaccine production (King *et al.,* 1981).

For immunoblotting (also known as western blotting), proteins separated by electrophoresis are transferred to a membrane (usually nitrocellulose) by diffusion or capillary flow, under vacuum or by electrophoresis. After a blocking step, in which nonspecific binding sites on the membrane are saturated with protein and/or detergent, the membrane is probed with a specific antibody, which may be a polyclonal serum or a MAb. Because the proteins have been denatured for electrophoresis, it can be expected that certain native epitopes, especially those dependent on protein conformation, will be destroyed and not detected. This is particularly relevant to the use of MAbs, which must be selected accordingly. Binding of antibody is visualised most commonly by an enzyme-substrate reaction. This may be achieved using an enzyme conjugated to a second antibody, a biotinylated-second antibody or a protein A conjugate. Alternative visualisation procedures can be used, included radioisotope labelling.

Immunoblotting is a highly discriminating procedure, since the immunological reactions seen can be identified with particular proteins. It can therefore provide particular information in relation to comparative results with different specimens and can avoid difficulties with non-specific reactions that may occur with alternative serological assays.

3.8.2 Application

3.8.2.1 Discrimination of FMD antibody produced by infection and by vaccination

In the epidemiological analysis and control of FMD in the field, there are benefits to determining whether a serological response in animals is the result of vaccination or infection. In particular, this applies in countries, which are free of FMD with vaccination, where it is important to monitor for the presence of any residual infection or new introduction of the disease.

Serological procedures are based on detection of antibody to FMD viral RNA polymerase or other non-structural proteins which are coded for by the virus but are generally absent, or present only in very low concentrations, in inactivated vaccines. Antibody to these proteins is therefore elaborated in response to infection but not to vaccination. Immunoblotting has been used to detect antibody to several bioengineered non-structural proteins of FMD virus (Bergmann *et al.*, 1993).

1. Bioengineered polypeptides designated 2C, 3A, 3B, 3ABC and 3D were purified, mixed and resolved on 12.5% SDS polyacrylamide gels.
2. The proteins were transferred electrophoretically to nitrocellulose membranes.
3. Membranes were probed with test serum samples and with positive and negative control sera.

A positive profile was one in which a serum reacted with all polypeptides. A negative profile had no reactivity and serum samples reacting with some but not all polypeptides were regarded as indeterminate. Serum samples from vaccinated animals all produced a negative profile Serum samples from cattle in FMD-free countries occasionally produced an indeterminate profile, with reactions to one or two antigens only. Indeterminate results were also occasionally obtained with samples from vaccinated cattle, but at a much lower rate that positive results with other serological assays.

3.9 Nucleic acid hybridisation and PCR techniques

3.9.1 Techniques

There are significant advantages to basing pathogen detection of the DNA or RNA. Successful bacterial or viral isolation is dependent on the presence of live pathogen in a specimen and is generally time consuming and expensive. It also requires the presence of live pathogen. Antigen detection procedures are limited by the amount and quality of antigen present in specimens. Nucleic acid is more resistant than protein to denaturation and can survive long periods of time (even centuries) in appropriate conditions. The limitation on nucleic acid detection has been the very small amounts that are available for detection. Notwithstanding, nucleic acid hybridisation techniques have been used to probe specimens, using a complementary strand of DNA or RNA, appropriately labelled – for example with an enzyme or a radioisotope. Specific base pairing produces a hybrid between the probe and the target, which can be detected appropriately. Nucleic acid probes have been developed and used for the detection of many pathogens.

However, the development of polymerase chain reaction (PCR) technology has revolutionised nucleic acid-based diagnostics and molecular research into infectious diseases. PCR is a means by which specific DNA sequences can be replicated *in vitro*. It can be applied to the preparation of material for basic studies and for preparing diagnostic reagents. It can also be applied to amplification of specific sequence present in a diagnostic specimen, so that it can then be detected by a variety of means. The principle of PCR can be summarised as follows:

1. Double stranded DNA is disrupted by heating to about 95°C.
2. The temperature is reduced to about 50°C and primers are annealed to the single stranded DNA. These are oligonucleotides (usually 20-30 base pairs in length) which are complementary to the 5′ region of the DNA and are required for initiation of DNA synthesis. Two oligonucleotides are used, each complementary to the positive or negative strand of the DNA and together flanking the region of the DNA to be amplified.
3. A DNA polymerase is added, together with deoxynucleotide triphosphates and the temperature is raised to about 70°C, under which conditions extension of the primers takes place to produce a complementary strand of DNA. The net result is two copies of the double stranded DNA, in place of the original copy.
4. The process is repeated cyclically, by raising and lowering the temperature, usually automatically in a thermal cycler. A thermostable polymerase is used (*Taq* DNA polymerase), which obviates the need to add more enzyme after each denaturing cycle. In principle, there is a doubling of the number of copies of the target sequence during each cycle, so that for example, one million copies can be generated over 20 cycles in a period of a few hours.
5. As a refinement to increase specificity, a second pair of primers can then be used, complementary to sequences already generated, to further amplify a smaller fragment of the DNA (*nested PCR*).
6. If the product is present in sufficient quantity, it can be seen by eye on a gel. For greater sensitivity and specificity, it is more common to identify the product by hybridisation with a labelled oligonucleotide probe. Finally, the product can be identified by direct sequencing.

Although systems have been described for RNA amplification, it is more common for RNA detection to be achieved by first transcribing a complementary DNA copy (cDNA), using an RNA-dependent DNA polymerase.

The application of PCR to disease diagnosis has been somewhat restricted to laboratories that have the required facilities, equipment, funding and expertise. The procedure must be undertaken in very clean conditions, since contamination with minute amounts of extraneous DNA may produce false positive results. Often this means that separate rooms and/or laminar flow cabinets must be used, with careful disinfection protocols to avoid cross-contamination. Equipment costs are high but will become justifiable to more laboratories as the range of applications increase. Methods are becoming better standardised so that training of staff in appropriate techniques can be rationalised. Certain standard reagents and consumables, such as *Taq* DNA polymerase, are expensive and not readily available in some countries.

The application of PCR (and other hybridisation techniques) to diagnosis is dependent on gene sequencing. Sequences must be targeted that are unique to the pathogen and the regions chosen for complementary primer production must be conserved within the genotypic range of the pathogen. The challenge then for many laboratories is access to specific primers and oligonucleotide detection probes. While these can be synthesised in suitably equipped laboratories, for most laboratories in developing countries there will be a dependence on having these reagents custom made by commercial sources or accessing them from international reference laboratories. Already, there is a growing level of support from such laboratories to introduce this technology into developing countries.

3.9.2 Applications

3.9.2.1 Detection of FMD virus by PCR

Antigen detection (by ELISA or CFT) is an adequate means of detecting FMD virus in epithelial samples from animals with unruptured or recently ruptured vesicles. At later stages of the disease, this becomes less reliable. For detection of virus in oesophageal/pharyngeal specimens from carrier animals, virus isolation is used, with its usual limitations. PCR was applied to the detection of FMD viral nucleic acid in such clinical specimens by Meyer *et al.* (1991). Primers flanking a conserved region of the polymerase gene were used, so that sequence to any of the virus types could be amplified. Product was detected by agarose gel electrophoresis, on the basis of molecular mass, with confirmation by hybridisation to a labelled probe. The procedure was specific for FMD viruses and at least as sensitive as alternative diagnostic procedures. Donn *et al.* (1994) also applied PCR to detecting FMD virus in oesophageal- pharyngeal tissues and fluids. They concluded that, although it was slightly more sensitive, at the current stage of development it was more suited to research than to routine diagnosis.

3.9.2.2 Diagnosis of CBPP by PCR

A PCR procedure has been developed to detect Mycoplasma DNA in pleural fluids from cattle with CBPP (Dedieu *et al.*, 1994). Two assays were used. The first detects a DNA sequence of about 460 base pairs from any member of the *Mycoplasma mycoides* cluster. The second PCR is specific for *Mycoplasma mycoides* subspecies *mycoides* S.C., the agent of CBPP. It detects a 275 base pair sequence within the original sequence, with three internal restriction sites producing a characteristic pattern on agarose gel electrophoresis. The sensitivity is such as to detect the equivalent of 100 colony-forming units of DNA. By using a dot-blot hybridization procedure for detection, in which a labelled probe is used, the sensitivity is increased to the equivalent of 1 colony-forming unit.

This procedure is currently in use in several African national veterinary laboratories.

3.9.2.3 PCR for detecting lumpy skin disease virus

The development of a rapid diagnostic test for lumpy skin disease (LSD) has been hindered by a number of factors. Electron microscopy is reliable but requires equipment that is not readily available in endemic areas. Also, LSD virus cannot be differentiated from another orthopoxvirus, which also produces skin lesions in buffalo. An antigen trapping ELISA is comparable to virus isolation in sensitivity but neither of them detects virus bound to neutralising antibody.

A sensitive and specific PCR was developed for the detection of capripox virus DNA in tissue culture supernatants and biopsy specimens (Ireland and Binepal, 1998). Two pairs of primers were used, complementary to gene sequences of the viral attachment and fusion proteins. Restriction endonuclease analysis of the products provided a simple means of confirming the identity of the PCR product. All reagents for the test are commercially available.

3.9.2.4 Detection of hog cholera virus in clinical specimens

Outbreaks of hog cholera can spread with alarming speed and early diagnosis is essential for control. Virus isolation takes several days and requires tissue culture facilities, including a reliable source of serum, free of both pestivirus and antibody. Staining of tissue sections from affected pigs is less sensitive and is not readily applied to large numbers of specimens. Detection of viral antigen by ELISA is more sensitive, can be applied to large numbers of specimens and usually demonstrates infection at the same time as the first clinical signs are occurring (Shannon *et al.*, 1993). Furthermore, use of MAbs in this assay can differentiate hog cholera viruses from other pestiviruses.

Harding *et al.* (1996) developed a reverse-transcriptase PCR procedure, which was applied to nucleic acid extracted from specimens. After two rounds of amplification, the assay was 100% sensitive and specific, in comparison to virus isolation. The authors used commercially available kits to extract RNA from specimens, analyse amplification product by electrophoresis and purify and measure DNA. Commercially available software was used to sequence nucleotides and develop phylogenic trees to compare virus strains.

3.9.2.4 Differential PCR assay for rinderpest and PPR

A reverse transcriptase method detects and differentiates between rinderpest and PPR viruses (Forsyth and Barrett, 1995). Viral RNA is transcribed to cDNA, which is then amplified using at least three primer sets. Two sets amplify regions of the fusion protein gene specific for either rinderpest or PPR viruses. The third set is based on a highly conserved region of the phosphoprotein gene, which will detect rinderpest and PPR viruses and other morbilliviruses. This is included to accommodate the possibility of a small change in the nucleotide sequence of the fusion protein producing a false negative result. The PCR products are resolved on an agarose gel. They are further identified by PCR using nested primer sets based on the amplified fusion protein sequences. Alternatively, the PCR products can be subjected to sequence analysis.

PCR can readily be applied to detection of rinderpest and PPR viruses in tears and swabs from eyes, mouth and gum erosions of affected animals. Such samples are readily obtained and easily transported to the laboratory. Furthermore, the PCR product can be used for sequence analysis for epidemiological studies, without the need to first isolate viruses in cell culture.

3.10 Nucleic acid analysis

3.10.1 Techniques

Genomic analysis of pathogens has been widely used to compare isolates. Fragments of DNA or RNA produced by nuclease digestion can be separated by electrophoresis to form bands whose position in a gel is dictated by molecular size. The patterns obtained for digests from different sources can be compared by running them in parallel. Greater discrimination can be obtained by running gels in two dimensions, under conditions producing separation in the first dimension on the basis of charge and in the second on the basis of size. Characteristic patterns are obtained (fingerprints) which can be compared visually. This has been used for comparing isolates of FMD virus (King *et al.*, 1981).

More meaningful analytical methods became available as the technology for sequencing nucleic acids developed. As sequence information became available, the true genotypic relationships between strains of a pathogen could be investigated and, by selecting appropriate parts of the genome, differences could be identified which related to differences in important epitopes. This has lead to the ability to construct phylogenic trees, which can give a graphic illustration of the relationships between a large number of strains.

3.10.2 Applications

3.10.2.1 Relationships between FMD virus isolates

The major immunogenic protein of FMD virus is VP1. When comparing sequences in the RNA coding region for VP1, aphthoviruses share about 40% nucleotide homology with cardioviruses and less with any other of the picornaviruses. Within the aphthovirus genus, there is at least 55% homology between all FMD types, with types A and C being more closely related to each other, as are types O and Asia 1, with the SAT viruses forming a separate group (Palmenberg, 1989).

Sequencing of key coding regions for VP1 is used to compare isolates for molecular epidemiological analysis. Differences demonstrated do not necessarily indicate antigenic differences that may be crucial, for example, in the prediction of cross protection from a particular field strain with a particular vaccine strain (Armstrong *et al.*, 1994). However, they are the best indicator of the genotypic relationships between isolates and permit studies to be undertaken on the evolution of strains within a geographic area, or the geographic movement of strains.

Sáiz *et al.* (1993) developed a phylogenic tree of FMD type O viruses based on VP1 sequences. They demonstrated four main lineages that largely correlated with the geographical origin of isolates. Two of these were isolates of European origin and one was an isolate of South American origin. The fourth lineage comprised isolates from North Africa and the Middle East, together with two European isolates, which may have been of non-European origin.
Kitching *et al.* used sequencing studies to trace the origins of several outbreaks of FMD (IAH, 1996). An outbreak of FMD virus type A in Albania in 1966 probably originated in India, spread to Saudi Arabia in imported livestock and to Albania, possibly directly from India or via Saudi Arabia, in contaminated meat products (Fig. 4). The same strain then spread to Macedonia. Outbreaks due to FMD virus type O in Greece, Bulgaria and Turkish Thrace were indistinguishable, implying that they were of a common origin. The illegal movement of animals was thought to be the most likely cause of the spread. In East Africa, field strains of several FMD virus types were indistinguishable from vaccine strains, raising the prospect of inadequate inactivation of vaccine. An isolate of FMD virus type SAT 2 from cattle in Zimbabwe was very closely related to isolates from buffalo on a nearby ranch and from wild populations from which the latter originated. (IAH, 1997). Isolates of FMD virus type O from pigs in Hong Kong, the Philippines, Taiwan province of China and Vietnam were closely related and it was thought that they probably had a common origin in China. These isolates were also highly adapted to pigs (Dunn and Donaldson, 1997).

Figure 4

Genetic relationships between FMD type A viruses

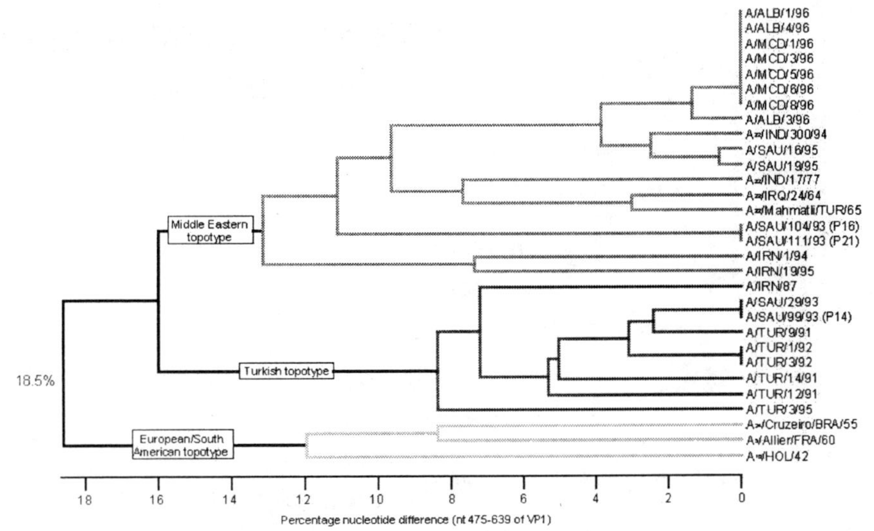

UPGMA dendrogram depicting the genetic relationships between foot-and-mouth disease type A viruses

(Ref. Knowles & Samuel, 1998)

3.10.2.2 Molecular epidemiology of rinderpest

Sequence analysis of part of the fusion protein gene of rinderpest viruses demonstrated distinct lineages, which reflected the geographical location of their isolation in Africa or Asia (Chamberlain *et al.*, 1993). Strains isolated from Kenya between 1987 and 1992 were closely related to isolates from Nigeria and Egypt in 1983/84. However, they were more distantly related to contemporary isolates from the Middle East and India and to older African isolates, including vaccine strains.

Between 1994 and 1996, disease was observed in wildlife in southern Kenya which was confirmed as rinderpest (Barrett *et al.*, 1998). The disease was seen mostly in national parks and in other areas where cattle were either vaccinated or not monitored due to their remoteness. The origin of the outbreak was therefore not immediately clear. RNA was purified from specimens, amplified by reverse-transcriptase PCR and DNA product was compared by sequence analysis with that from earlier and contemporary virus isolates. This revealed that the wildlife isolates were all of common origin and most related to a giraffe isolate from 1964 and other African isolates from the 1950s and 1960s. These strains were designated Africa type 2, being a different lineage to later African isolates, which were, designated Africa Type 1 (Fig. 5). A further lineage, Asia, was represented by recent isolates from that region. It appears, therefore, that two distinct lineages of African isolates have co-existed in equatorial Africa for over 30 years.

These studies have important implications for the Global Rinderpest Eradication Programme. It was previously believed that only one endemic focus of rinderpest virus remained in Africa, centred around the borders of Kenya, Uganda, Ethiopia and Sudan. The emergence of disease caused by a virus of a second lineage raises concerns about the effectiveness of surveillance methods, which were largely predicated on the assumption that a recrudescence of disease would be detected by overt disease in cattle.

Figure 5

Phylogenetic relationships of rinderpest virus strains

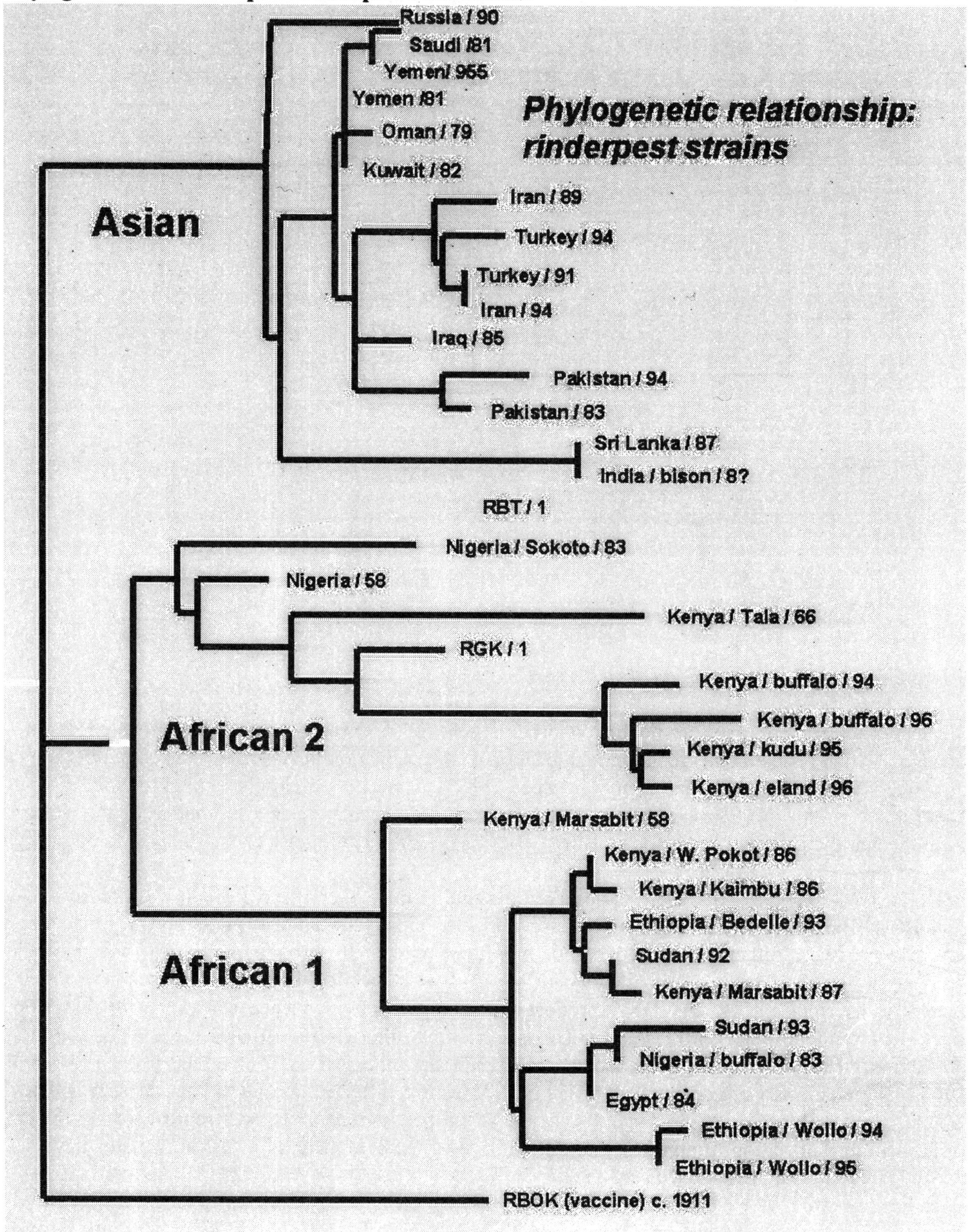

(Ref. Barrett *et al.*, 1998)

3.11 Diagnostic challenges for BSE

While several transmissible spongiform encephalopathies (TSEs) have been known for many years, the identification of bovine spongiform encephalopathy (BSE) as a new disease became one of the most important transmissible disease issues in recent times. The important issues included the very size of the epidemic in the United Kingdom, its main (or only) means of transmission by ingestion of ruminant-derived meat meal, its apparent ability to affect a range of hosts, including antelope and cats as well as cattle and ultimately, the evidence that the same agent was apparently responsible for a variant form of Creutzfeld-Jakob disease (vCJD) in humans.

Diagnosis was primarily on the basis of clinical signs and characteristic histological lesions in the brains of affected animals. These lesions were consistent with those in other species affected with TSE but in the case of cattle were remarkably uniform in location and consistency, to the extent that microscopic examination of one section of medulla oblongata at the level of the obex is sufficient for a diagnosis to be made (Taylor, 1996). This suggests that in BSE, there is only one strain of the infectious entity. Fibrils can be detected by electron microscopy and these comprise an abnormal protease-resistant form (PrP^{Sc}) of a normal host protein (PrP^{C}), which survives autolysis and can therefore be detected in tissues unsuitable for histopathology.

The basis of infectivity of BSE (and other TSEs) has not been established but may be PrP^{Sc} (the prion theory) or may in addition involve an informational molecule (the virino theory). If the former is the case, it is difficult to explain strain variation in scrapie. If the latter is true, then no such molecule has been identified (Taylor, 1996). Since the alteration of PrP^{C} is a post-translational event, there is nothing at the nucleic acid level that can be identified with disease. Also, there is no immune response to PrP^{Sc}, although it can be identified by immunoblotting using antiserum raised in rabbits and a monoclonal antibody that specifically detects the altered protein has been developed (Korth *et al.*, 1997). In at least some forms of scrapie, PrP^{Sc} can be found in lymphoreticular tissues prior to the onset of clinical disease but this has not been possible in BSE. Two proteins identified as members of the 14-3-3 family have been associated with clinical CJD and BSE (Lee and Harrington, 1997), although they may not be of value for establishing a diagnosis in early symptomatic cattle (Robey *et al.*, 1998).

Thus there are still difficulties in understanding the nature of the infectivity of TSEs and in confirming a diagnosis in clinical cases, without recourse to slaughter of the suspect animal. The BSE epidemic is clearly coming to an end but differential diagnosis will be a continuing concern for many years to come.

3.12 Appropriate technology

Laboratories will vary in the technology that they can apply to disease diagnosis. They may be limited by equipment, by funds available for purchasing consumables and by staff expertise. An international reference laboratory will generally have access to and be actively involved in development of the latest techniques. It should also be in a position to provide advice on techniques and to supply specific reagents to other laboratories. In developing countries in particular, decisions often need to be made at the national level as to what kind of laboratory expertise and technology is appropriate and sustainable.

It is important that diagnosticians should not be afraid to embrace new technology but at the same time should recognise their own constraints in introducing it. It is usually not the technology itself but the support that is required that dictates how readily a new assay can be introduced. The pen-side test for rinderpest is the easiest diagnostic test to use but represents on the the most sophisticated technologies. Conversely, virus isolation represents 'old' technology but is one of the most challenging capabilities to maintain.

ELISA kits that contain all required ingredients, including specific reagents can be used in any laboratory that has the basic microtitration equipment. A national laboratory that anticipates undertaking large numbers of tests may elect to have more automated equipment, but should be very careful about becoming dependent on equipment that is difficult to service locally. Most important of all is adequate quality control. This requires attention to such detail as recycling plasticware and to availability of specific reagents. It is a big commitment for a laboratory to opt for an assay for which it must prepare its own antigens or antisera. In particular, any district or regional laboratory in a country should be able to access all required consumables from its national laboratory. The FAO/IAEA Joint Division sponsors projects in which essential ELISA equipment and technical support is provided to laboratories for specific diagnostic activities for its priority diseases.

Nucleic acid diagnostic technologies are at the point that ELISA technology reached about 20 years ago. In principle, some PCR assays for which reagents can be obtained commercially or from reference laboratories, can be performed in a laboratory that has a thermal cycler and standard electrophoresis equipment. The expertise to undertake this new technology is less widespread and this will be a major limiting factor in the adoption of PCR for routine diagnosis. However, the other limitation will be the cost of consumables, which are generally much greater than for serological procedures.

In general, new technologies should not be adopted just because they are new. There must be clear justification in terms of cost savings or significantly improved diagnostic capability. Thus, there is not a strong argument for replacing antigen detection ELISAs for FMD or rinderpest with PCR assays. On the other hand, PCR may be a very worthwhile approach to CBPP diagnosis in the later stages of an eradication campaign, where rapid and definitive decisions on individual cases are important. The FAO/IAEA is promoting the application of PCR technologies to the major transboundary diseases and such sponsorship would be an ideal way for developing countries to develop the required expertise.

References

Armstrong, R.M., Samuel, A.R., Carpenter, W.C., Kant, R. & Knowles, N.J. 1994. a comparative study of serological and biochemical methods for strain differentiation of foot-and-mouth disease type A viruses. *Vet. Microbiol.*, **39**: 285-298.

Barrett, T., Forsyth, M.A., Inui, K., Wamwayi, H.M., Kock, R., Wambua, J., Mwanzia, J. & Rossiter, P.B. 1998. Rediscovery of the second African lineage of rinderpest virus: its epidemiological significance. *Vet. Rec.*, **142**: 669-671.

Bergmann, I.E., Augé de Mello, P., Neitzert, E., Beck, E. & Gomes, I. 1993. Diagnosis of persistent aphthovirus infection and its differentiation from vaccination response in cattle by use of enzyme-linked immunoelectrotransfer blot analysis with bioengineered nonstructural viral antigens. *Amer. J. vet. Res.*, **54**: 825-831.

Chamberlain, R.W., Wamwayi, H.M., Hockley, E., Shaila, M.S., Goatley, L., Knowles, N.J. & Barrett, T. 1993. Evidence for different lineages of rinderpest virus reflecting their geographic isolation. *J. Gen. Virol.*, **74**: 2775-2780.

Davidson, F.L., Crowther, J.R., Nqindi, J., Knowles, N.J., Thevasagayam, S.J. and Van Vuuren, C.J. 1995. Antigenic analysis of SAT 2 serotype foot-and-mouth disease virus isolates from Zimbabwe using monoclonal antibodies. *Epidemiol. Infect.*, **115**: 193-205.

Dedieu, L., Mady, V. & LeFevre, P.C. 1994. Development of a selective polymerase chain reaction assay for the detection of *Mycoplasma mycoides* subsp. *mycoides* S.C. (contagious bovine pleuropneumonia agent). *Vet. Microbiol.*, **42**: 327-339.

Donn, A., Martin, L.A. & Donaldson, A.I. 1994. Improved detection of persistent foot-and-mouth disease infection in cattle by the polymerase chain reaction. *J. Virol. Meth.*, **49:** 179-186.

Dunn, C.S. & Donaldson, A.I. 1997. Natural adaptation to pigs of a Taiwanese isolate of foot-and-mouth disease virus. *Vet. Rec.*,**141**: 174-175.

Ferris, N.P. 1988. Selection of foot and mouth disease antisera for diagnosis by ELISA. *Rev. sci. tech. Off. int. Epiz.*, 7: 331-346.

Ferris, N.P. & Dawson, M. 1988. Routine application of enzyme-linked immunosorbent assay in comparison with complement fixation for the diagnosis of foot-and-mouth disease and swine vesicular disease. *Vet. Microbiol.*, **16**: 201-209.

Forsyth, M.A. & Barrett, T. 1995. Evaluation of a polymerase chain reaction for the detection and characterisation of rinderpest and peste des petits ruminants for epidemiological studies. *Virus Res.*, **39**: 151-163.

Harding, M.J., Prud'homme, I., Gradil, C.M., Heckert, R.A., Riva, J., McLaurin, R., Dulac, G.C. & Vydelingum, S. 1996. Evaluation of nucleic acid amplification methods for the detection of hog cholera virus. *J. Vet. Diagn. Invest.*, **8**: 414-419.

Heller, C., Stem, C., Wamwayi, H. & Grieve, A. 1998. Development of a filter paper-based ELISA for rinderpest antibodies. *Vet. Rec.*, 142: 729.

IAH. 1994. BBSRC Institute for Animal Health: Annual Report.

IAH. 1995. BBSRC Institute for Animal Health: Annual Report.

IAH. 1996. BBSRC Institute for Animal Health: Annual Report.

IAH. 1997. BBSRC Institute for Animal Health: Annual Report.

Ireland, D.C. & Binepal, Y.S. 1998. Improved detection of capripoxvirus in biopsy samples by PCR. *J. Virol. Meth.*, **74**: 1-7.

Kendal, C., Ionescu-Matiu, I. & Dreesman, G.R. 1983. Utilization of the biotin/avidin system to amplify the sensitivity of enzyme-linked immunosorbent assay (ELISA). *J. Immunol. Methods*, **56**: 329-339.

King, A.M.Q., Underwood, B.O., McCahon, D., Newman, J.W.I. & Brown, F. 1981. Biochemical indentification of viruses causing the 1981 outbreaks of foot and mouth disease in the UK. *Nature*, **293**: 479-480.

Knowles, N.J. & Samuel, A.R. 1998. Molecular techniques in foot-and-mouth disease epidemiology. In: *Towards Livestock Disease Diagnosis and Control in the 21st Century*. Proc. Intnl. Symposium on Diagnosis and Control of Livestock Diseases. FAO/IAEA, Vienna, April 1997, pp. 185-201.

Korth, C., Stierli, B., Streit, P., Moser, M., Schaller, O., Fischer, R., Shulz-Schaeffer, W., Kretzschmar, H., Raeber, A., Braun, U., Ehrensperger, F., Hornemann, S., Glockshuber, R., Riek, R., Billeter, M., Wüthrich, K. & Oesch, B. 1997. Prion (PrP^{Sc})-specific epitope defined by a monoclonal antibody. *Nature*, **390:** 74-77.

Lee, K.H. & Harrington, M.G. 1997. 14-3-3 and BSE. *Vet. Rec.*, **140**: 206-207.

Le Goff, C. & Thiaucourt, F. 1998. A competitive ELISA for the specific diagnosis of contagious bovine pleuropneumonia (CBPP). *Vet. Microbiol.*, **60**: 179-191.

Libeau, G., Diallo, A., Colas, F. & Guerre, L. 1994. Rapid differential diagnosis of rinderpest and peste des petitis ruminants using an immunocapture ELISA. *Vet. Rec.*, **134**: 300-304.

Meyer, R.F., Brown, C.C., House, C., House, J.A. & Molitor, T.W. 1991. Rapid and sensitive detection of foot-and-mouth disease virus in tissues by enzymatic RNA amplification of the polymerase gene. *J. Virolog. Meth.*, **34**: 161-172.

OIE. 1996. Manual of Standards for Diagnostic Tests and Vaccines. 3rd ed. Office International des Epizooties, Paris, France.

Palmenberg, A.C. 1989. Sequence alignments of picornaviral capsid proteins. In: Molecular Aspects of Picornaviral Infection and Detection. Semler, B.L. and Ehrenfeld, E. (eds.). American Society for Microbiology, Washington, USA. pp. 211-241.

Paweska, J.T., Barnard, B.J.H. & Williams, R. 1995. The use of sucrose-acetone extracted Rift Valley fever virus antigen derived from cell culture in an indirect enzyme-linked immunosorbent assay and haemagglutination-inhibition test. *Onderst. J. Vet. Res.*, **62**: 227-233.

Price, C.P. & Newman, D.J. (eds.). 1997. Principles and practice of immunoassay. Second ed. Macmillan Reference Ltd., London.

Robey, W.G., Jackson, R., Walters, R.L., Brackett, J.M., Harrington, C.A. & Killian, W.R. 1998. Use of cerebrospinal fluid levels of 14-3-3 in predicting neurodegeneration in confirmed BSE symptomatic cattle. *Vet. Rec.*, **143**: 50-51.

Roeder, P.L. & Le Blanc Smith, P.M. 1987. The detection and typing of foot-and-mouth disease virus by enzyme-linked immunosorbent assay: a sensitive, rapid and reliable technique for primary diagnosis. *Res. Vet.Sci.*, **43**: 225-232.

Rweyemamu, M.M. 1984. Antigenic variation in foot-and-mouth disease: studies based on the virus neutralization reaction. *J. Biol. Stand.*, **12**: 323-337.

Sáiz, J.C., Sobrino, F. & Dopazo, J. 1993. Molecular epidemiology of foot-and-mouth disease virus type O. *J. Gen. Virol.*, **74**: 2281-2285.

Saiki, R.K., Gelfand, D.H., Stoffel, S., Scharf, S.J., Higuchi, R., Horn, G.T., Mullis, K.B. & Erlich, H.A. 1998 . Primer-directed enzymatic amplification of DNA with a thermostable DNA polymerase. *Science*, **239**: 487-491.

Shannon, A.D., Morrissy, C., Mackintosh, S.G. & Westbury, H.A. 1993. Detection of hog cholera virus antigens in experimentally-infected pigs using an antigen-capture ELISA. *Vet. Microbiol.*, **34**: 233-248.

Singh, G. & Singh, I. 1997. Use of dot-immunobinding assay for visual detection of rinderpest antibodies in vaccinated cattle. *Trop. An. Hlth. Prodn.*, **29**: 73-76.

Taylor, D.M. 1996. Bovine spongiform encephalopathy – the beginning of the end? *Br. Vet. J.*, **152:** 501-518.

Towbin, H. & Gordon, J. 1984. Immunoblotting and dot immunobinding – current status and outlook. *J. Immunol. Methods*, **72**: 313-340.

Woodbury, E.L., Samuel, A.R., Knowles, N.J., Hafez, S.M. & Kitching, R.P. 1994. Analysis of mixed foot-and-mouth disease virus infections in Saudi Arabia: prolonged circulation of an exotic serotype. *Epidemiol. and Infect.*, **112**: 201-211.

Zola, H. (ed.). 1995. Monoclonal antibodies: the second generation. BIOS Scientific Publishers, Oxford, UK.

Chapter 4

Advances in Vaccine Technology

4.1 Introduction

New technology in vaccine production is directed toward improving the immunogenicity and safety of vaccines, their shelf life and their cost of production. Descriptions of current vaccine technology and issues related to the quality control of vaccines are provided in another FAO publication (Mowat and Rweyemamu, 1997). This chapter is directed toward new developments that are largely the outcome of the application of recombinant DNA technology. The benefits are only just starting to be realised but there is no doubt that, as with diagnostic technology, we are at the start of a revolution.

Vaccines have conventionally been live or inactivated pathogens. Live viruses are generally economical to produce, because only a small amount needs to be inoculated into the host, with subsequent replication producing the antigenic mass required for a satisfactory immune response. Also, replication results in appropriate antigen presentation for stimulation of humoral and cell-mediated immune mechanisms. However, there are also constraints in their use. There is always a risk of contamination with adventitious agents. There are circumstances in which suitable vaccine strains, which are not too virulent, cannot be developed or dissemination of the vaccine virus is undesirable. Inactivated vaccines may then be used. These are nearly always more expensive as larger amounts of antigen must be administered to the host. Often an adjuvant is required to enhance immunogenicity of the antigen and in any event, often the response is essentially humoral only. Both live and inactivated vaccines can degrade in unsuitable environmental conditions, especially at high ambient temperatures. Maintenance of vaccine quality to the point where it is administered to the host, is a major challenge.

4.2 Recombinant DNA technology

Recombinant DNA technology has provided the tools to enable us to better understand the structure and function of pathogens. It has allowed us to construct variants with reduced pathogenicity or greater stability, rather than seeking to attenuate strains by empirical means. We are able to isolate particular proteins of known importance in stimulating a protective immunity and to produce them in novel host systems in greater purity and at often enormous cost savings. These are the main subjects of the discussion below, which is illustrated by examples of vaccine development for the major transboundary diseases. With the exception of CBPP, the diseases being considered are viral and this will therefore be the emphasis of this chapter

Because this technology is central to much of the discussion, the principles involved are briefly outlined here. For additional detail, there are many reference texts, of which Old and Primrose (1994) is an excellent example. The essential steps are:

1. Nucleic acid is extracted from the target pathogen and digested with restriction endonucleases.
2. Fragments are separated on the basis of their molecular mass, usually on an agarose gel.
3. Isolated fragments are incorporated into a vector – the process of *gene cloning*. This enables the DNA to be amplified so that sufficient material is available for analysis. Typically, the cloning vector will be a plasmid or phage with known characteristics and incorporated into a transformed *E. coli*. If the source is an RNA virus, the RNA must first be transformed into complementary DNA (cDNA).

4. Recombinants are screened or selected. Vectors carry a selectable marker, such as antibiotic resistance, that can be used to identify the presence of the vector. In the case of a phage, this can be done on the basis of plaque formation. Selection for the presence of the foreign gene may be by direct detection of the gene, such as by DNA hybridisation, or by detection of the gene product as an antigen, using specific antibody. Since many clones may need to be screened, an efficient screening strategy must be determined in advance.
5. The gene can now be sequenced. A common method is the dideoxy procedure. Nucleotide analogues are progressively incorporated into a DNA chain during replication and terminate the growth of the chain at that point. Chains of varying length are generated and gel electrophoresis is then used to identify the sequence of the nucleotides. Some of the sequencing procedure has been automated and it is possible to perform all of the steps so far by a combination of PCR for amplification (even if the sequence is partly unknown), followed by automatic sequence analysis.
6. The functional part of the DNA sequence can then be incorporated into an *expression vector* for generation of the product. It may use existing promoter to drive the expression or a foreign promoter may also be inserted. The vector will usually need to be elaborated in a eukaryotic system, for complete expression of the product – for example, for glycosylation of proteins. It may be a yeast (which can be readily grown *in vitro*), a baculovirus (which can be grown to high titre in the host insect or insect tissue culture) or a mammalian virus, which is grown in cell culture. Alternatively, a bacterial or virus vector may be inoculated directly into the final host, to achieve immunisation against the target pathogen.

4.3 Modified live virus vaccines

In the past, attenuation of a virus, to produce a strain of reduced pathogenicity as a candidate for a live vaccine, was undertaken empirically, usually be multiple passage in an abnormal host. Thus for example, rabies vaccines were produced by passage a virus in embryonating eggs to a low or high passage level, depending on the degree of attenuation sought. There was no guarantee whether or when sufficient attenuation would be achieved or whether the resulting virus would still be immunogenic. There was also concern that the virus might revert to full virulence on passage through the normal host, when applied as a vaccine.

The application of molecular technologies has produced a greater understanding of the molecular basis for the pathogenicity of organisms. We can identify the genetic changes required for reduced pathogenicity and then manipulate the genome by a variety of processes to make the change.

4.3.1 Application

4.3.1 1.A gene-deleted Aujeszky's disease vaccine

The first veterinary application of a deletion mutant vaccine was the production of attenuated vaccines for Aujeszky's disease (Binns, 1993). Viruses were deficient in the thymidine kinase gene, a deletion too large to be retrieved by mutation. Some also have gene deletions for non-essential glycoproteins. This enabled antibody responses in animals infected with vaccine or wild viruses to be differentiated, a valuable characteristic for epidemiological studies and in situations where eradication is the goal.

4.4 Synthetic peptides as vaccines

Modern methods in molecular biology and immunology have enabled us to identify the sites on viruses where the binding of antibodies occurs that are responsible for the neutralisation of infectivity. As sequence information became available, the prospect arose of producing peptides that would mimic these epitopes in stimulating an antibody response that would provide protective immunity. Such an approach could enable stable and completely defined immunogens to be manufactured chemically. Attempts were made to immunise animals against FMD virus, using peptides corresponding to sequences of the VP1 protein, which constitutes the major immunogenic site of the virus. Guinea pigs were protected by immunisation with a peptide of 19 amino acids (Bittle *et al.*, 1982) and Di Marchi *et al.* (1986) demonstrated protection in cattle with a peptide representing two separate regions of the VP1 protein. However, protection required a large amount (more than one milligram) of the peptide, even though a strong antibody response was achieved with much lower amounts. This suggest that successful immunisation with peptides may require T cell as well as B cell recognition. Although the approach has not yet met with success, it may do so when the interactions of B and T cell epitopes are better understood (Brown, 1997).

4.5 Sub-unit vaccines

Immunisation with live virus vaccines is generally the easiest and most efficient form of achieving a protective immunity. The main benefit of inactivated vaccines is that they are safer, but their production is far more expensive, as a larger mass of virus must be produced. Improper inactivation of vaccines has been a significant concern with FMD and it is well established that it has resulted in outbreaks of the disease. The goal of sub-unit vaccines is to target certain immunogenic fragments of the virus that can be produced by a more efficient process and are at no risk of carrying infectious virus.

The desired gene or genes are inserted into an efficient expression vector. A favoured one is baculovirus. Baculoviruses infect insects and produce intranuclear inclusions, the major component of which is a virus-encoded protein, polyhedrin (Old and Primrose, 1994). This is not essential for replication and its gene can be replaced by foreign one driven by the same very strong promotion system to express the new protein as up to 50% of the cell protein. Production may be conducted in insect cell culture or using the insects themselves – for example, silkworms, whose culture is well established in the silk industry.

4.5.1 Applications

4.5.1.1 Immunisation against African swine fever

It has proved notoriously difficult to immunise against African swine fever (ASF). Neutralising antibodies cannot be detected after infection. However, infection with an attenuated strain confers protection and immunity can be passively transferred with serum. The mechanisms for protection are not well understood.

Part of the virus glycoprotein that is responsible for haemagglutination of pig erythrocytes in vitro, has sequence similarities to a T cell adhesion receptor (Ruiz-Gonzalvo *et al.*, 1996). The gene was amplified by PCR, cloned and sequenced. A recombinant baculovirus was constructed which expressed the haemagglutinin of ASF virus. Pigs inoculated with baculovirus infected cells survived challenge with virulent ASF virus.

4.5.1.2 Immunisation against bluetongue with virus-like particles

Isolated, monomeric sub-units of a virus are generally not highly immunogenic and a variety of strategies are employed to overcome this. Pearson and Roy (1993) co-infected cells with two recombinant baculoviruses, producing together two capsid proteins and two core proteins of bluetongue virus. The expressed proteins self-assembled into virus-like particles which were immunogenic in sheep.

4.6 Improved vaccine formulation and antigen presentation

Maximisation of an immune response is usually dependent to a greater or lesser extent on stimulation of both humoral and cell-mediated immunity. B cells recognise linear and conformation determinants of native antigen through their surface immunoglobulin (Rimmelzwaan and Osterhaus, 1997). However, for T cell recognition, proteolytic degradation to peptides in antigen-producing cells must first take place, the peptides then associating with major histocompatibility complex (MHC) molecules. Two different pathways, exogenous and endogenous, have been identified, with presentation to T helper and cytotoxic T cells respectively.

Adjuvants are used to enhance the immune response to an antigen, by acting as an immunostimulant or by improving antigen presentation. They are more commonly used for inactivated vaccines, where it is more difficult to achieve an adequate immune response. This problem is increased with sub-unit vaccines and has led to an increasing interest in adjuvants.

The form of antigen presentation has an important effect on immune stimulation. Antigens incorporated into liposomes or into immune stimulating complexes (ISCOMs), appear to be highly immunogenic. ISCOMs are a structures formed by saponin and cholesterol in which protein antigens are embedded. They appear to stimulate both humoral and T cell responses and have been used in producing protective immunity to enveloped viruses in at least eight different virus families (Hughes and Babiuk, 1994).

Mineral adjuvants have a depot effect, which results in a slow release of antigen from an inflammatory focus. Aluminium hydroxide is the most widely used compound and is generally effective and safe. Oil adjuvants are often more effective, but need to be formulated as emulsions, with water as the continuous phase, to obtain a liquid of low viscosity that can be readily inoculated.

Sometimes bacterial extracts are included, such as heat-killed mycobacteria in Freund's complete adjuvant, or muramyl dipeptide, which is the smallest active component from this extract (Horzinek *et al.*, 1997).

4.6.1 Applications

4.6.1.1 An ISCOM vaccine against CBPP

Conventional vaccines for contagious bovine pleuropneumonia (CBPP) employ live organisms administered by subcutaneous inoculation. Among difficulties that are encountered, in the fact that the more highly immunogenic vaccines are also less attenuated and severe vaccine reactions can occur. Strain $T_1/44$ and its streptomycin-resistant variant T_1-SR are the currently recommended strains (OIE, 1996). In any event, immunity is of short duration. Inadequate quality control in vaccine production and lack of a good cold-chain to the field have both caused live vaccines to perform poorly (Tulasne *et al.*, 1996). Oil adjuvanted vaccines have been developed (Garba *et al.*, 1986) but not tested extensively.

An ISCOM vaccine prepared from detergent-solubilised cells of *Mycoplasma mycoides* subspecies *mycoides* SC produced strong and long lasting humoral and cell-mediated immune responses (Abusugra, *et al.*, 1997). It is possible that such a vaccine may represent an attractive alternative if subsequent larger scale experiments verify its performance.

4.6.1.2 Emergency vaccines for FMD

With successful eradication of FMD from many countries, increasing consideration has been given to contingency plans for the event of an outbreak in a susceptible population of livestock. Although slaughter of affected herds is the first option, many countries have elected to include emergency ring vaccination as an alternative, if rapid spread appears likely. An International Vaccine Bank has been established from which member countries can draw vaccine in an emergency.

Vaccine is formulated as required, using concentrated inactivated FMD viral antigen stored over liquid nitrogen. It must be suitable for use in all species and be readily formulated. Most importantly, it must be capable of inducing a rapid immunity, to protect inoculated animals and to limit dissemination of the virus. This is particularly important in the case of pigs, because they excrete very large amounts of FMD virus in aerosols and are often a major source of disease spread.

Work by Doel *et al.* (1994) showed that conventional vaccines adjuvanted with aluminium hydroxide/saponin or with oil, protected cattle as early as four days after vaccination but that pigs were only protected 21 to 28 days after vaccination. Experiments were conducted with novel oil adjuvants, Montanide ISA 25 and 206, the first of which forms an oil-in-water emulsion and the second, a water-in-oil-in-water emulsion (Salt *et al.*, 1998). The vaccines had a low viscosity and did not produce the local reactions at the inoculation site often experienced with conventional oil emulsion vaccines. Pigs were protected from challenge as early as four days after vaccination. This was not always associated with detectable levels of neutralising antibody and it may be that the stimulation of cell-mediated immune mechanisms is particularly important in this early protection. Pigs challenged seven days after immunisation did not excrete sufficient virus to infect susceptible pigs in contact. FMD vaccines formulated with these adjuvants clearly have a good potential for containing outbreaks of disease in an emergency situation.

4.7 Chimeric live vaccines

Genes coding for key proteins of the target pathogen can be inserted into a virus, which is infective for the host animal and can safely be used as a vaccine. The principle combines the benefits of traditional live and inactivated vaccines:

- immunogenic sites of the pathogen are presented to the host immune system by a means in which a protective immune response is stimulated
- relatively small volumes of vaccine can be produced, as the chimeric virus will replicate in the host to produce the required antigenic mass
- there is no risk of reversion to virulence of the pathogen, as only a small portion of it is presented.

A virus vector must be chosen that can support the insertion of adequate amounts of foreign gene and this is normally a virus with a relatively large genome. Candidate vectors include adenoviruses, herpesviruses and poxviruses. The vector must replicate in the host animal, at least to the extent that expression of the gene insert takes place. The vector should grow readily in cell culture. Poxviruses have received particular attention as candidate vectors. They have the potential for multiple insertions to immunise against two or more pathogens at the one time. They are also heat stable. Furthermore, they can be very readily grown. Vaccinia virus can be grown by scarification of the abdomen of a calf, producing over 200,000 vaccine doses from one animal.

Because the serological response in respect to the target pathogen is limited to that against the inserted gene product, the use of recombinant vaccines permits differential serology, that can discriminate vaccination from infection. This property can be used to advantage for epidemiology studies and disease control activities.

While vaccinia virus is an excellent candidate, concerns over potential pathogenicity for humans has required the selection of stable attenuated strains for use as vectors (Yamanouchi *et al.*, 1998).

Alternatives to vaccinia virus include avian poxviruses, which readily infect mammalian cells and express inserted genes but do not undergo replication in mammalian tissue.

4.7.1 Applications

4.7.1.1 A recombinant vaccine for rabies

The first such vaccine to be developed and used was a vaccinia virus recombinant with the glycoprotein gene of rabies virus inserted. This vaccine has been effective in controlling fox rabies in Europe, by incorporating the virus into baits. The virus survived well in the baits, despite wide temperature variations, including freezing and thawing (Brouchier *et al.*, 1996). The virus has also been used in the United States of America for controlling rabies in raccoons and coyotes. The recombinant vector carries a gene for tetracycline which produces a band in the teeth of bait recipients. This is a valuable means of monitoring bait uptake.

With the reluctance to use vaccinia viruses as vectors for human immunisation, an alternative was sought. A recombinant canary pox virus carrying the rabies glycoprotein gene is immunogenic in several mammalian species, including humans (Fries *et al.*, 1996.)

4.7.1.2 Protection against Newcastle disease with recombinant viruses

On a worldwide basis, Newcastle disease is one of the most important epidemic diseases, causing losses in commercial farms and village chickens. Inactivated vaccines are generally expensive to produce and administer but are used where the spread of live virus is undesirable or to overcome maternal immunity. Live vaccines of varying virulence are used and the more virulent ones are generally also more immunogenic.

A variety of recombinant viruses have been constructed. A recombinant attenuated fowlpox virus, expressing both the haemagglutinin-neuraminidase and the fusion proteins of Newcastle disease virus has been shown to confer immunity to both fowlpox and to Newcastle disease (McMillen *et al.*, 1994). It is licensed in the USA and marketed commercially.

Herpesvirus of turkeys, the virus commonly used for vaccination of chickens for Marek's disease, has also been used as a vector. A recombinant expressing the fusion protein of Newcastle disease virus produced protection against Newcastle disease as well as Marek's disease (Morgan *et al.*, 1992).

The potential application of this technology in the developing world needs to be considered in the context of alternative solutions. Thermostable live Newcastle disease vaccines can be produced on a cottage industry scale at very low cost, making the vaccine widely available in developing countries (Spradbrow and Copland, 1996). However, intensive poultry producers administer vaccines for a range of diseases, mostly viral. There is the potential for recombinant fowlpox viruses, to provide multivalent protection against several diseases with one vector (Boyle and Heine, 1993).

4.7.1.3 Concurrent protection against Aujeszky's disease and hog cholera

The thymidine-kinase gene-deleted virus used for Aujeszky's disease vaccination has also been used as a vector. Insertion of a glycoprotein gene from hog cholera virus protected pigs against both diseases (Van Zijl *et al.*, 1991).

4.7.1.4 Recombinant vaccines for rinderpest

The conventional attenuated live virus rinderpest vaccine has most of the desirable characteristics of a good vaccine. It is easy and economical to grow in cell culture, it confers immunity to all strains of the virus, and induces a prolonged immunity after one vaccination. Several poxvirus recombinant vaccines have been developed and the benefit is simply their thermostability. In the freeze-dried form they not do require a cold-chain. Given the enormous challenges involved in distribution of vaccine for the Global Rinderpest Eradication Programme, almost all in developing countries, the assurance of vaccine potency at the point of use is a major benefit.

Recombinant vaccinia viruses containing either or both of the genes for rinderpest virus haemagglutinin (H) or fusion protein (F) produced protection against challenge in cattle (Tsukiyama, *et al.*, 1989; Giavedoni *et al.*, 1991; Inui, *et al.*, 1995). They also protect goats against challenge with PPR virus (Romero *et al.*, 1995). Capripox viruses have also been used as vectors and have the additional benefit of conferring protection against lumpy skin disease. A recombinant capripox virus carrying the genes for the F and H proteins of rinderpest virus produced complete or partial protection against challenge for up to 12 months after vaccination (Ngichabe, *el al.*, 1997). However, pre-existing immunity to lumpy skin disease interfered with successful immunisation with this vaccine.

4.8 DNA vaccines

An exciting development in vaccine technology is the prospect of using naked DNA as a vaccine. Inoculation of DNA into muscle results in the expression of proteins in the muscle cells and the potential for producing a protective immunity to a range of pathogens has been demonstrated. The DNA can also be administered percutaneously using a gene gun which fires DNA-coated gold microparticles and permits the use of less than 1 μg of DNA (Ramsay *et al.*, 1997a).

Advantages of the approach include the purity, stability and simplicity of production of plasmid DNA (Ramsay *et al.*, 1997a). Genes expressing antigens of different strains of a pathogen or of different pathogens could be included. Indeed, a broad protection across strains of influenza virus was demonstrated using the nucleoprotein gene, which induced a strong cytotoxic T-lymphocyte response in mice (Ulmer *et al.*, 1993). It appears that expressed antigen is in the native form and is therefore optimally presented to, and processed by, the immune system.

The DNA persists for up to 18 months and it has been speculated that it is continuously expressed (Yamanouchi *et al.*, 1998) and re-immunisation can be undertaken by the same means with no inhibition by pre-existing antibody. In another approach, primary immunisation with DNA was followed by boosting with a recombinant virus vector (Ramsay *et al.*, 1997b).

Concerns about the integration of foreign DNA into the host genome may be a major obstacle for the application of this technology in humans, but the implications are not as great for livestock. Mice were protected against rabies challenge by immunisation with 2 μg of DNA on gold particles, delivered with a gene gun (Lodmell *et al.*, 1998), with a subsequent booster. Protective immunity lasted for more than 300 days.

4.9 The role of cytokines

Cytokines modulate the immune response by acting as intercellular messengers of differentiation, proliferation and/or activation of the cells responsible for immune function (Pasquini *et al.*, 1997). Different sub-sets of T helper cells produce more than 20 interleukins and other cytokines and accessory molecules that stimulate or suppress cell-mediated or humoral immune mechanisms.

The prospect has been explored of improving the immune response to an antigen by using the appropriate cytokines. The most attractive avenue is to incorporate a gene into a DNA vaccine. The approach has been demonstrated in immunisation against hepatitis B and hepatitis C (Pasquini *et al.*, 1997). However, there are constraints, in particular because prolonged expression of cytokine genes could produce unwanted immunological or haemopoietic side effects. Another practical problem is that many of the cytokines are highly species-specific in their activity, so that application of the technology to livestock species is likely to be some years away.

References

Abusugra, I., Wolf, G., Bölske, G., Thiaucourt, F. & Morein, B. 1977. ISCOM vaccine against contagious bovine pleuropneumonia. 1. Biochemical and immunological characterization. *Vet. Immunol. Immunopathol.*, **59**: 31-48.

Bittle, J.L., Houghten, R.A., Alexander, H., Shinnick, T.M., Sutcliffe, J.G. & Lerner, R.A. 1982. Protection against foot-and-mouth disease by immunization with a chemically synthesized peptide predicted from the viral nucleotide sequence. *Nature*, **298**: 30-33.

Boyle, D.B. & Heine, H.G. 1993. Recombinant fowlpox virus vaccines for poultry. *Immunol. Cell Biol.*, **71**: 391-397.

Brouchier, B., Aubert, M.F.A., Pastoret, P.-P., Masson, E., Schon, J., Lombard, M., Chappuis, G., Languet, B. & Desmettre, Ph. 1996. Field use of a vaccinia-rabies recombinant vaccine for the control of sylvatic rabies in Europe and North America. *Rev. Sci. Tech. Off. Int. Epiz.*, **15**: 947-970.

Brown, F. 1997. In: *Vaccine Manual: The production and quality control of veterinary vaccines for use in developing countries.* Mowat, G.N. & Rweyemamu, M.M. eds. FAO, Rome, Italy.

DiMarchi, R., Brooke, G., Gale, C., Cracknell, V., Doel, T. & Mowat, N. 1986. Protection of cattle against foot-and-mouth disease by a synthetic peptide. *Science*, **232**: 639-641.

Doel, T.R., Williams, L. & Barnett, P.V. 1994. Emergency vaccination against foot-and-mouth disease: rate of development of immunity and its implications for the carrier state. *Vaccine*: **12**: 592-600.

Fries, L.F., Tartaglia, J., Taylor, J., Kauffman, E.K., Meignier, B., Paoletti, E. & Plotkin, S. 1996. Human safety and immunogenicity of a canarypox-rabies glycoprotein recombinant vaccine: an alternative poxvirus system. *Vaccine*, **14**: 428-434.

Garba, S.A., Ajayi, A., Challa, L.D., Bello, M.K., Gazama, J.N.Z., Gimba, H., Ngbede, J., Bitrus, B. & Adeoye, A.O. 1986. Field trial of inactivated oil-adjuvant Gladysdale strain vaccine for contagious bovine pleuropneumonia. *Vet. Rec.*, **119**: 376-377.

Giavedoni, L., Jones, L., Mebus, C. & Yilma, T. 1991. A vaccinia virus double recombinant expressing the F and H genes of rinderpest virus protects cattle against rinderpest and causes no pock lesions. *Proc. Natl. Acad. Sci. USA.*, **88**: 8011-8015.

Horzinek, M.C., Schijns, V.E.C.J., Denis, M., Desmettre, P. & Babiuk, L.A. 1997. In: *Veterinary Vaccinology.* P.-P. Pastoret, J. Blancou, P. Vannier & C. Verschueren, eds. Elsevier, Amsterdam, The Netherlands. pp 131-152.

Hughes, H.P.A. & Babiuk, L.A. 1994. In: *Modern Vaccinology.* E. Kurstak, ed. Plenum Publishing Corporation, New York, USA. pp 87-118.

Inui, K., Barrett, T., Kitching, R.P. & Yamanouchi, K. 1995. Long-term immunity in cattle vaccinated with a recombinant rinderpest vaccine. *Vet. Rec.*, **137**: 669-670.

Lodmell, D.L., Ray, N.B. & Ewalt, L.C. 1998. Gene gun particle-mediated vaccination with plasmid DNA confers protective immunity against rabies virus infection. *Vaccine*, **16**: 115-118.

Morgan, R.W., Gelb, J., Schreurs, C.S., Lütticken, D., Rosenberger, J.K. & Sondermeijer, P.J.A. 1992. Protection of chickens from Newcastle and Marek's diseases with a recombinant herpesvirus of turkeys vaccine expressing the Newcastle disease virus fusion protein. *Av. Dis.*, **36**: 858-870.

Mowat, G.N. & Rweyemamu, M.M. (eds.). 1997. *Vaccine Manual: The production and quality control of veterinary vaccines for use in developing countries.* FAO, Rome, Italy.

Ngichabe, C.K., Wamwayi, H.M., Barrett, T., Ndungu, E.K., Black, D.N. & Bostok, C.J. 1997. Trial of a capripoxvirus-rinderpest recombinant vaccine in African cattle. *Epidem. Infect.*, **118**: 63-70.

OIE. 1996. Manual of Standards for Diagnostic Tests and Vaccines. 3rd ed. Office International des Epizooties, Paris, France.

Old, R.W. & Primrose, S.B. 1994. Principles of gene manipulation: an introduction to genetic engineering. 5th ed. Blackwell Science Ltd, Oxford.

Pasquini, S., Xiang, Z., Wang, Y., He, Z., Deng, H., Blaszczyk-Thurin, M. & Ertl, H.C.J. 1997. Cytokines and costimulatory molecules as genetic adjuvants. *Immunol. Cell Biol.* **75**: 397-401.

Pearson, L.D. & Roy, P. 1993. Genetically engineered multi-component virus-like particles as veterinary vaccines. *Immunol. Cell Biol.*, **71**: 381-389.

Ramsay, A.J., Ramshaw, I.A. & Ada, G.L. 1997a. DNA immunization. *Immunol. Cell Biol.*, **75**: 360-363.

Ramsay, A.J., Leong, K.H. & Ramshaw, I.A. 1997b. DNA vaccination aginst viral infection and enhancement of antiviral immunity following consecutive immunization with DNA and viral vectors. *Immunol. Cell Biol.*, **75**: 382-388.

Rimmelzwaan G.F. & Osterhaus, A.D.M.E. 1997. The immune response. In: Ve*terinary Vaccinology*. P.-P. Pastoret, J. Blancou, P. Vannier & C. Verschueren, eds. Elsevier, Amsterdam, The Netherlands. pp55-67.

Romero, C.H., Barrett, T., Kitching, R.P., Bostock, C. and Black, D.N. 1995. Protection of goats against peste des petitis ruminants with recombinant capripoxviruses expressing the fusion and haemagglutinin protein genes of rinderpest virus. *Vaccine*, **13**: 36-40.

Ruiz-Gonzalvo, R., Rodrigeuz, F. & Escribano, J.M. 1996. Functional and immunological properties of the baculovirus-expressed hemagglutinin of African swine fever virus. *Virology*, **218**: 285-289.

Salt, J.S., Barnett, P.V., Dani, P. & Williams, L. 1998. Emergency vaccination of pigs against foot-and-mouth disease: protection against disease and reduction in contact transmission. *Vaccine*, **16**: 746-754.

Spradbrow P.B. & Copland, J.W. 1996. Production of thermostable Newcastle disease vaccines in developing countries. *Prev. Vet. Med.*, **29**: 157-159.

Tsukiyama, K., Yoshikawa, Y., Kamata, H., Imaoka, K., Asano, K., Fananhashi, S., Maruyama, T., Shida, H., Sugimoto, M. & Yamanouchi, K. 1989. Development of heat-stable recombinant rinderpest vaccine. *Arch. Virol.*, **107**: 225-235.

Tulasne, J.J., Litamoi, J.K., Morein, B., Dedieu, L., Palya, V.J., Yami, M., Abusugra, I., Sylla, D. & Bensaid, A. 1996. Contagious bovine pleuropneumonia vaccines: the current situation and the need for improvement. *Rev. Sci. Tech. Off. Int. Epiz.*, **15**: 1373-1396.

Ulmer, J.B., Donnelly, J.J., Parker, S.E., Rhodes, G.H., Felgner, P.L., Dwarki, V.J., Gromkowski, S.H., Deck, R.R., DeWitt, C.M., Friedman, A., Hawe, L.A., Leander, K.R., Martinez, D., Perry, H.C., Shiver, J.W., Montgomery, D.L. & Liu, M.A. 1993. Heterologous protection against influenza by injection of DNA encoding a viral protein. *Science*, **259**: 1745-1749.

Yamanouchi, K., Barrett, T. & Kai, C. 1998. New approaches to the development of virus vaccines for veterinary use. *Rev. Sci. Tech. Off. Int. Epiz.*, **17**: 641-653.

van Zijl, M., Wensvoort, G., de Kluyver, E., Hulst, M., van der Gulden, H., Gielkens, A., Berns, A. & Moormann, R. 1991. Live attentuated pseudorabies virus expressing envelope glycoprotein E1 of hog cholera virus protects swine against both pseudorabies and hog cholera. *J. Virol.*, **65**: 2761-2765.

Appendix I

Technology at Work

A Detailed Case Study on the Application of Technology in the Fight Against Rinderpest and Peste des Petits Ruminants (PPR), Major Transboundary Animal Diseases

1. The availability of technology

Diseases need to be controlled and if possible, eradicated. Technologies assist in the fulfilment of these objectives. The skill of the day is in matching the appropriate technology to the job to be undertaken. Transboundary diseases affect both developed and developing economies. By and large developed livestock economies are those that have never suffered from, or have long since eradicated, or can afford to stamp out, the more infectious and pathogenic transboundary animal diseases. The same economies provide the engine for further development aimed at improving diagnostic and vaccine technology in order to curb those diseases that do still cause them problems. In contrast, livestock industries in the world's least developed economies still suffer from a crippling array of animal diseases for most of which they lack the technological means of control, the resource base to afford new innovations or if available, the means to means of implementation. In essence then transboundary diseases are controlled by developed economies and not controlled by poorly developed economies; intermediate situations exist.

In spite of the existing constraints, veterinary services around the world share a common desire to improve the global environment within which livestock live so that, as and when the means to control or even eradicate a transboundary disease become technically or politically feasible, appropriate control or eradication schemes are launched. Unfortunately, where it universally desirable to control or eradicate a pathogen occurring in a least developed country (LDC), the pace of progress is determined very largely by the availability of external funding resources. Under these circumstances such programmes will involve the co-operation between donors and local veterinary managers. These persons must take joint responsibility for the selection of the current technologies most appropriate to the task. Donors have the added responsibility of ensuring the existence of objective review processes to allow progress to be properly gauged and to accept the need to allow innovative ideas and technologies to be incorporated where they offer a more rational use of limited resources. Managers should therefore maintain a constant awareness of technological advances and assess whether their potential strategic values outweigh those in current use.

For the second half of the twentieth century veterinarians around the world have been attempting to make the eradication of rinderpest the first successful example of the elimination of an animal pathogen. The end of this process is palpably close, and yet new problems have arisen that may still throw into doubt much of what has been achieved. Many of the difficulties concerning the correct choice, application and management of diagnostic and vaccine technologies are exemplified within the current Global Rinderpest Eradication Programme (GREP). This section will examine these issues in depth using other disease situations where they provide additional supporting to a particular discussion point.

Before a disease can be eradicated there must exist a sound understanding of its natural survival mechanisms. This can only be gained through a constant studying the agent within the livestock population within which it is being maintained. It is essential to understand how the agent is being transmitted in order to propose a strategy which will interrupt this transmission. This calls for the continual application and refinement of technologies which support the diagnosis and differential diagnosis of the agent, the continuing study of its pathogenesis and means of transmission, serological techniques to facilitate geographic survey work, vaccine technology and serological techniques to assist in the management of vaccination campaigns. To the extent that the application of these technologies contributes to a knowledge of the epidemiology of the agent, and because microbiological agents are adaptable and able to change, the key to moving from control to eradication lies in the constant applied research as a means of keeping abreast of changing field situations and mechanisms for undertaking technical reviews of control strategies and appropriate supporting technologies.

2. The techniques for studying the epidemiology of a transboundary disease taking rinderpest as a case study

Rinderpest is regarded as being an acute viral disease of bovines and of a number of wildlife species within the order *Artiodactyla.*. The FAO is currently co-ordinating a Global Rinderpest Eradication Campaign (GREP) for which the currently scheduled completion date is 2010. It is becoming increasingly clear that achieving this objective will be more complicated than was expected. Over the last 40 years the classic technologies, including uncomplicated diagnostic methods, sound virus isolation techniques and an effective vaccine, appeared to have made possible the realisation of this dream. In the last decade however, problems have arisen which would have eventually proved insoluble were it not for the ability to gain new insights into the current behaviour of the virus through the use molecular epidemiological methods. Even so, it is not clear whether we fully understand to what extent this virus has been able to adapt itself to persist in the face of high levels of immunity within the livestock population in which it occurs.

In as much as part of this adaptation might consist of a reduction in virulence in situations of endemicity and high vaccine coverage, and periodic recrudescence to a more virulent form when large susceptible populations become available, it is necessary to attempt to develop a better understanding of the adaptive changes the virus has undergone. To do this we have to attempt to follow possible earlier developments in persistently endemic situations and how this may still affects us at the present time. In all of this it may be necessary to develop a better understanding of the mechanisms of viral virulence, a subject on which we are still ignorant. It remains to be seen if eradication can be successfully completed without this information.

3. Virulence as an epidemiological marker

3.1 The development of low virulence strains in the field

Because samples are frequently submitted from rinderpest outbreaks associated with severe disease and high mortality laboratory collections usually contain a preponderance of highly virulent strains, i.e. viruses which give high (≥70%) case fatality rates on re-inoculation into experimental animals. This situation has led to the assumption that rinderpest virus strains are always highly virulent in nature whereas in fact the reverse is more probably the norm. The more we examine endemic field situations the more we can find evidence that in them the virulence of the virus diminishes with time.

In Tanzania, where rinderpest has probably been endemic for almost a century, strains with differing levels of innate virulence co-circulated for a number of years (Branagan and Hammond, 1965) and the strain that survived the longest appears to have been the one with the lowest level of virulence. From a background in which the virus was disseminated over large tracts of the country in the early years of the present century, and caused outbreaks involving large numbers of cattle, evidence of a diminishing virulence gradually emerged. Given that attenuated vaccines were yet to be developed, in the initial stages of control considerable attention was given to measures aimed at quarantining infected herds. Even though hyperimmune serum was used within these herds, recorded herd mortality rates probably gave some measure of the virulence of the virus involved. In the years from 1921 to 1926 the observations shown in Table 1 were made.

Table 1. Mortality rates in quarantined cattle herds in Tanzania.

Year	no. outbreaks	no. cattle involved	mortality rate
1921	86	124,597	?
1923	93	374,000	11.4%
1925	86		9.3%
1926	43	150,870	4.3%

As it is clear that rinderpest entered Tanzania in a highly virulent form as part of the great African panzootic of the late 19th century, these observations suggest that 30 years later the virulence of some strains was considerably reduced. Additional evidence comes from the recorded occurrence of "very mild rinderpest" at Tabora in the centre of the country in 1926. Over the next few years further evidence accrued suggesting the persistence of strains of rinderpest which were milder than had been considered normal. Thus in 1933 two outbreaks were noted in Lake Province which were said to be both mild and atypical. In 1934 outbreaks around Singida were mild and a clinical diagnosis was apparently difficult to make. In 1937 the situation in the southern highlands was said to be exacerbated by the mildness of the disease which thereby became well established before it was recognised. In 1944 mild clinical outbreaks around were again recorded around Tabora. Still in East Africa, Plowright (1998) reminds us that reports of similar variations in virulence were not unknown in Kenya and that the Masai people were wont to deliberately spread mild strains among their young cattle.

Although it seems clear that the virulence of the virus was being modified, it is also apparent that this was a gradual rather than an abrupt process. Thus in 1936 when the virus entered a herd of totally susceptible zebu cattle a mortality rate of 20% was recorded. It is probably also worth recalling the observation of Maurer et al (1955) that individual animals vary widely in resistance to rinderpest and that strain characteristics should be based on a number of observations; also that most strains of the virus produce less severe lesions in young stock than in adults. This suggests that just because a strain appears to be mild in calves, it was not necessarily mild for adults bearing out the observation from a 1951 Annual Report describing the disease as being generally insidious in calves and only flaring up in non-immune adults.

Although Lowe et al., (1947), isolated a bovine rinderpest strain characterised by low mortality, the presence of mouth lesions and the absence of diarrhoea, it was Robson et al., (1959) who isolated the first well characterised mild strain of the virus. The isolate in question came from a sick Eland (*Taurotragus oryx*) found on the Ol Balbal plains in northern Tanzania. On reference to experimental cattle a zero mortality rate was recorded, both in East African zebu and East African grade cattle. In zebu cattle only 3/17 exhibited mild changes in the oral cavity whereas with grade cattle mouth lesions were seen in 21/21 animals (suggesting that there were minor variations in innate resistance between the two breed types). In respect of other virulence parameters (incubation period, maximum temperature, duration of pyrexia & development of diarrhoea) the experimental animals behaved homogeneously. What was striking about this virus was the mildness of the infectious episode. Although the virus was readily transmissible to other cattle, its virulence did not increase over nine serial passages in cattle. Sheep and goats were both susceptible to parenteral inoculation and developed pyrexia unaccompanied by any other signs. With the isolation of this virus it was finally clear that field selection pressures alone could produce a "mild" but transmissible strain of rinderpest which did not kill its host.

In 1960-61 Plowright isolated five very similar strains of rinderpest from northern Tanzania and three from southern Kenya. Given that strains with a high virulence for cattle could still be encountered in northern Kenya, what was difficult to appreciate at the time was that high virulence strains had ceased to exist in Tanzania. In fact so well adapted had rinderpest become that it was able to persist in northern Tanzania from 1962 to 1965 without its presence being detected. Not surprisingly then, the last rinderpest strain isolated from Tanzania in 1966 was shown to be mild in experimental cattle (Macadam, 1968). The technology underpinning the isolation, characterisation and preservation of such viruses consisted of cell cultures, susceptible experimental cattle and lyophilisation.

3.2 Attenuating selection pressures

Given that cattle are the natural hosts for rinderpest virus, it can be readily attenuated by propagating it in a number of atypical hosts (embryonated eggs, rabbits, goats, cell cultures). It is clear therefore, that under the influence of the correct selection pressure or pressures, the virulence of the virus can be greatly reduced. Generally in the laboratory this process is seen as the selective survival and overgrowth of a series of spontaneously occurring mutants of decreasing virulence; what is not so clear in nature is exactly what constitutes the selection pressure. In the Tanzanian situation, because of the relative frequency with which game animal species became infected, some authors postulated that they were involved in selecting attenuated variants but others thought that they might actually enhance the virulence for cattle.

On the other hand it seems equally likely that in any long-term endemic situation, a high proportion of the adult bovine population will be immune and that, compared to a fully susceptible population, this will decrease the rate at which infected and susceptible hosts come into close contact and this in turn diminishes the chance of contact transmission. Under these circumstances, strains of rinderpest which do not kill their host and which may be excreted over longer periods are likely to predominate. In Tanzania for the first 50 years of endemicity, rinderpest was faced with a mixture of herds with either low or high levels of immunity, depending on whether they had been involved in a recent outbreak or not. After 1940, with the introduction of mass vaccination campaigns, a higher all-round level of immunity would have prevailed. It is suggested that these were, at least in part, the circumstances responsible for the selection of strains of rinderpest with low virulence and a high probability of survival within vaccinated populations. The continued success of such strains would lie in the fact that within a partially vaccinated population their continued existence could never be excluded on clinical grounds alone.

3.3 The danger of reversion to virulence

In the only example available, the genomic length of the virulent and attenuated variants of the Kabete "O" strain of rinderpest were essentially the same. It is therefore impossible to envisage attenuation as a process of accumulating deletion mutations and in theory it must be assumed that if confronted with the correct selection pressure mild strains could regain their virulence. Large susceptible cattle populations might constitute just such a pressure and once reversion started, it would be understandable if more rapidly transmitting viruses, with shorter excretion periods and greater pathogenic potential were selected, and gave rise to epidemics of the disease. It can now be suggested that reduced virulence evolves during pastoral endemicity but virulence is regained when the virus is transferred into a new population with homogeneously low herd immunity levels, and in which it has the possibility of rapid transmission. Such a more virulent variant might ultimately self-extinguish or persist, depending on its rate of contact with fresh susceptible hosts. However, even if this phenomenon is of a temporary nature, the original mild strain may still be present within the population and re-emerge when the virulent virus has run its course. We now have an insight into how, by diminishing in virulence, rinderpest developed a survival strategy that may yet cause a series of novel problems to those attempting to eradicate it.

4 Pathology as an indicator of virulence

4.1 The pathology of rinderpest

Using classic histopathological techniques, Maurer (1955) showed that rinderpest attacks the epithelium of the digestive tract where it produces early and characteristic lesions. In the stratified squamous epithelium of the mouth, necrotic lesions commence in the deeper layers of the stratum malpighii, just above the basal layer, the virus having been carried there haematogenously. Foci develop, consisting of growing numbers of infected cells with pyknotic and fragmented nuclei and with eosinophillic cytoplasm. These cells become separated from adjoining healthy cells but do not form into a vesicle. The further recruitment of surrounding cells increases the size of the necrotic lesion extending it towards the surface where it produces a slight elevation to the cornified layer, macroscopically visible as a tiny greyish-white, slightly elevated puncta. Subsequent coalescence and enlargement of these necrotic foci may be accompanied by detachment of the debris leaving a shallow erosion on the surface of the mucus membrane, bounded by normal epithelium and having sharply demarcated margins. As the basal layer is rarely penetrated, even though the underlying capillaries make them look red and raw, they are essentially non-haemorrhagic.

In the abomasum and intestines, necrosis of the single layered columnar epithelium exposes the underlying vascular system leading to capillary haemorrhage in the underlying lamina propria. In the abomasum the pyloric region is the most severely and consistently involved with microscopic foci of necrosis accompanied by capillary congestion and haemorrhage in the underlying lamina propria. The lesions tend to follow the edges of the plicae which are highly coloured between red and brown, becoming slate-grey in more long-standing cases. The columnar epithelium of the small intestine is less frequently involved.

In the large intestine the ileocaecal valve and surrounding mucosae show necrosis and erosion of the epithelium and congestion and haemmorhage of the underlying lamina propria. In well developed cases the crests of the folds of the mucous membrane throughout the caecum are bright red due to the presence of petechiae which can be so numerous that they resemble diffuse haemorrhages. Microscopically however, these lesions are distended capillaries within the lamina propria. The distribution of the congestion along the crests of the folds of the mucosae gives rise to a "zebra striped" appearance. Similar pathology extend through the colon and rectum.

Rinderpest virus also has an affinity for lymphoid tissue, where its effect is to produce lymphocyte necrosis. Microscopically, this is strikingly evident in the spleen, lymph nodes and Peyer's patches. The number of lymph follicles involved depends on the severity and stage of the disease. These changes are accompanied by capillary congestion and oedema, but only the oedema is grossly visible. If the loss of lymphoid tissue is severe the follicles are transformed into fibrillar, acellular matrices surrounded by plasma cells, nuclear debris and numerous macrophages. Capillary endothelia are usually unaffected, and congestion and haemorrhage are conspicuously absent. Because of their exposed position, the entire lymphoid contents of Peyer's patches may slough to leave a deeply cratered intestinal wall.

4.2 Rinderpest pathogenesis

These findings were later complemented by the quantitative pathogenesis studies of Liess & Plowright (1964), Plowright (1964) and Taylor & Plowright (1965). These studies demonstrated that virulent rinderpest entered a host through the epithelium of the upper or lower respiratory tract, infected and multiplied in the nearest drainage lymph node, developed a viraemia and was haematogenously distributed to, and multiplied in, lymphoid tissues and the mucous membranes of the respiratory and intestinal tracts. Coincident with the viraemia, virus could be detected in the urine, faeces and nasal excretions. In contrast, Taylor et al. (1965) showed that a strain of the virus attenuated to the point where it ceased to be transmissible, retained the capacity to replicate in lymphoid tissues but had lost the ability to replicate in epithelial tissues. It would seem from these studies that to some extent virulence is determined by the virus' tissue tropisms.

Using an immunohistochemical (peroxidase anti-peroxidase) technique, Wohlsein et al. (1993 & 1995) were able to correlate the severity of the clinical disease, the extent of morphological lesions and the distribution of viral antigen in tissues; in their studies mild, virulent and per-acute strains of the virus were used. For all strains, antigen was closely associated with mucosal lesions, however animals infected with the per-acute Saudi strain 1/81 strain showed multiple, partly coalescing clusters of antigen containing cells in the mouth, abomesum, duodenum, jejunum, ileum and large intestine, and single clusters of antigen staining cells in the oesophagus, reticulum and rumen; lymphoid tissues were also heavily involved. Viral antigen was also present in the salivary glands, bile duct epithelia and in hepatocytes. In the lungs it was present in airway epithelia, interstitial lymphocytes, alveolar macrophages and alveolar lining cells. In the kidneys cells of the renal pelvis were involved while in the eye viral antigen was observed in the conjunctiva. With the acute RGK/1 strain, similar changes were seen in the digestive tract and lymphoid tissue but lymphocyte infiltration of the sub-epithelial connective tissue was reduced, as was involvement of parenchymatous organs. Both acute and per-acute viruses were detected in the same type of cells in the different organs however, there were marked differences in the amount of antigen present.

4.3 Rinderpest virulence

In comparison with West Pokot/86/1, a comparatively mild strain, animals infected with the acute RGK/1 showed significantly higher numbers of antigen containing cells in all affected tissues. In the oral cavity RGK/1 infected cells throughout the stratum spinosum but with West Pokot, antigen distribution was extremely focal and limited. Similarly, in the abomasum numerous antigen bearing lymphocytes, macrophages, fibroblasts and endothelial cells were found in the lamina propria of an RGK/1 infected steer whereas they were very much fewer in number with West Pokot. RGK/1 infected cells were present in moderately high amounts in the white pulp of the spleen, and in follicular and paracortical areas of the lymph nodes. With West Pokot antigen was confined to follicular areas and was absent from the spleen.

From these studies it is possible to conclude that virulence is directly correlated with the distribution and rate of replication in the host tissues and that strains with the ability to generalise beyond than the digestive tract and lymphoid tissues cause the rapid death of the host. Mild strains which seldom cause the death of the host still affect the target tissues but give rise to limited cell destruction and are less invasive than more virulent strains. Under laboratory conditions strains can be modified to the point where the ability to replicate in lymphoid tissues is retained but the ability to replicate in the cells of surface epithelia is lost; such strains can be used as a vaccine. While investigating the mechanics of virulence, these studies shed no light on the underlying molecular events. They did however demonstrate that variations in virulence are part of a continuous spectrum related to variations in the range of cells attacked and the rapidity of replication within a particular cell type.

5 Techniques for virus diagnosis

5.1 Immunodiffusion tests

The classic rinderpest diagnostic technique is based on visualising a precipitation reaction between rinderpest antigens and immunoglobulins in an agar substrate. The test can be undertaken using passive diffusion of the reagents, as in an agar-gel immunodiffusion technique, or active diffusion as in an immunoelectrophoresis test (Foreman et al., 1983). Although these are very robust tests they do require the use of a potent and specific rinderpest immune serum. In general it is difficult to develop such a serum in bovines and the customary source of hyperimmune serum is the rabbit inoculated with the Nakamura III strain of lapinised rinderpest. Unfortunately it is becoming increasingly difficult to obtain this virus as a result of which modified antiserum production methods have multiplied. A number of these seem to induce antibodies to bovine serum albumen which produces non-specific test reactions and in consequence, false positive results. Another factor that now detracts from the value of this test is that a rinderpest hyperimmune serum will react with antigens of Peste des Petits Ruminants (PPR) virus. Should the disease for which diagnostic confirmation is being sought be associated with bovines, it is probably safe to assume that it is rinderpest. However, should the disease have occurred in a small ruminant, it is more likely to have been PPR.

5.2 Improved diagnostic and differential diagnostic techniques for local use

It is of course important that Veterinary Services maintain an awareness of the extent of their exposure to both rinderpest and PPR viruses as in fact a growing number of countries are simultaneously infected or at risk to infection with both viruses. Under these circumstances epidemiological features should be taken into account if a disease from which morbillivirus antigens are demonstrated is encountered.. For instance the presence of clinical disease in sheep and goats but not in contact cattle is more compatible with a diagnosis of PPR than of rinderpest while disease in cattle but not in small ruminants is more compatible with a diagnosis of rinderpest. However, in the final analysis it is possible for rinderpest to affect small ruminants and it is apparent that PPR is transmissible to large ruminants may also affect a minority of individuals with a clinical disease (El Hag Ali, 1973, Govindarajan et al., 1997/8).

In a number of African and Asian countries, even though the incidence of rinderpest is declining, it will continue to be important to be able to obtain a valid differential diagnosis between PPR and rinderpest at a local level. Within GREP there is a requirement that once a country considers itself free of clinical rinderpest and is prepared to support this view by ending all anti-rinderpest vaccination, all clinical outbreaks of rinderpest-like disease must be subject to a differential diagnosis. In a number of these countries, the last decade has seen the realisation that both PPR and rinderpest were affecting the national livestock industries at the same time. As PPR in small ruminants can certainly be regarded as a rinderpest-like disease, a requirement emerged for a robust test which would differentiate these two diseases. This was provided by a differential immunocapture ELISA test. In principle the sample to be analysed is first allowed to react with the detection antibody and the immunocomplex formed is captured by a second antibody previously adsorbed onto the surface of an ELISA plate. In the test system described by Libeau et al, (1994) viral specific immunocomplexes were formed with monoclonal antibodies to non-overlapping domains of the viral nucleocapsid protein and captured by a third monoclonal antibody recognising an epitope common to the nucleocapsid proteins of both rinderpest and PPR. This test has been introduced throughout the state disease investigation laboratories in India where it has been widely used to confirm the diagnosis of PPR in sheep and goats. It is proving to be a relatively easily transferred technology.

In 1997 field trials were undertaken with a chromatographic strip test, a so called "pen side rinderpest diagnostic test" for the rapid detection of the presence of rinderpest antigens which are known to be present in ocular secretions. This test is based on the activation, specific binding and migration of coloured microspheres along a disposable cellulose acetate strip. The test result can be developed within a few minutes in the field or in the veterinary investigation laboratory, and is so simple and so rapid that its acceptability as a test will be overwhelming. In addition to its usefulness in veterinary investigation work, it would seem to be a particularly appropriate test for undertaking security control tests for consignments of animals moving between administrative regions of a possibly infected country.

5.3 Reference laboratory tests

Reference laboratories may be expect calls to provide a differential diagnosis of transboundary diseases in critical situations and often, with poor specimens. These considerations suggest the need for improved diagnostic tests based on the application of molecular biological techniques. Nucleic acid hybridisation is a very specific technique for the identification of pathogenic viruses. High sensitivity of detection can be achieved either on extracted nucleic acid material or *in situ* on histological sections. The technique is based on the ability of any nucleic acid to bind in a very stable, hydrogen bonded duplex structure to its complementary sequence. Such a duplex is more stable and specific than an antigen-antibody complex and, depending on the stringency with which the reaction is carried out, can be made to detect either the exact complementary sequence or one closely related to it. DNA probes to the N genes of rinderpest and PPR are now available and can be used to identify and differentiate between the two viruses (Diallo et al., 1989).

The presence of rinderpest virus in formalin fixed tissues may be detected using a digoxigenin-labelled riboprobe to a segment of the genome for the N protein (Brown, 1997). The test results indicated that clear and distinct signals could be obtained from a variety of rinderpest-infected tissues. This technique should be routinely available at reference laboratory level with a view to attempting to transfer the technology to sub-reference disease investigation laboratories.

The reverse transcription polymerase chain reaction has proved a very powerful tool in rinderpest diagnosis and can be used to differentiate rinderpest from PPR. As a technique RT/PCR has found a ready application at the reference laboratory level, but non-specific products can occasionally be produced and the specificity of the DNA product should always be checked independently, preferably with a labelled oligonucleotide probe. These considerations lead to the conclusion that at the present time the RT/PCR technique should be retained at the level of the national or international reference laboratory.

5.4 The need for virus isolation

At one time virus isolation was an important component of virus diagnostic procedures and could be undertaken in a number of national reference laboratories. Increasingly, it is a procedure that is being discarded due to the need for complicated and lengthy laboratory procedures, skilled manpower and adequate laboratory budgets. It may seem that if we have the ability to determine the entire genetic sequence of a virus we must be privy to everything there is to know about it in which case there would seem to be no need to continue to actually isolate the virus from the field. One of the advantages of the RT/PCR technique is that it may succeed in providing diagnostic information even if the entire virus is no longer present. One of its disadvantages (in relative terms) is that sequence it produces is not that of the entire virus. Nevertheless, from time to time it is important to look at the entire virus. It might for instance be necessary to look at the nucleic acid sequence of other parts of the virus, but most importantly it may be vital to understand the virulence profile of a particular strain. Unfortunately for most viruses this information still cannot be derived from sequence analysis. Virus isolation therefore remains an important procedure in the diagnosis of rinderpest and one which we ignore at our peril. Teams undertaking investigations into the possible presence of rinderpest should bear in mind at all times that once a virus is isolated, in depth studies can be undertaken to determine its genotype, phenotype and relationship with other isolates, all of which is information vital to an understanding of the epidemiology of the virus. Therefore every possible effort should be made to retrieve samples from the field and submit them to a reference laboratory in good condition within a cold chain. In the last few years the track record of isolating rinderpest viruses has been poor.

The standard operating procedure for teams undertaking an investigation should include the availability of modules of a rapid diagnostic test and transport containers for collecting specimens for virus isolation. As a contingency measure, formol saline containers should be included in order to fixing tissues for *in situ hybridisation*. From the number of recent occasions when vital information has not been retrieved from the field, it is clear that training in the application of these techniques is a further requirement.

6. Molecular epidemiology

6.1 Sequence analysis

Of course the main advantage of the RT/PCR technique over DNA probe analysis is that the resulting DNA can be sequenced and the data analysed at the genetic level to determine the relationship between the virus in question and previous isolates. This is a very powerful tool and it allows us to draw conclusions which, until a few years ago, would have been very difficult to make. Whether this new-found wisdom will ultimately assist us in our attempts to control and eliminate pathogenic micro-organisms remains to be seen.

In essence, sequence analysis is able to tell us where a virus may have come from, revealing that a new virus may have entered the population within which it is already represented. This may lead us to previously unsuspected portal of entry, or to conclude that we have been misconstruing the apparent absence of the virus.

6.2 Phylogenetic lineages of rinderpest

In 1994 rinderpest appeared in wild buffaloes and kudu in Tsavo National Park in southern Kenya in an outbreak which persisted into 1995 and re-appeared in Nairobi National Park in 1996 in buffalo and eland. (Barrett et al., 1998). Initial concern centred on the fact that the original outbreak might have been diagnosed five months earlier than it actually was and that in consequence emergency responsiveness had not as good as it could have been. As the origins of the outbreaks could not be back-traced with any degree of certainty it was assumed that the virus had been introduced by cattle and that the virus must have originated in eastern Uganda or southern Sudan where virulent strains of the virus were known to exist.

RNA was purified from post-mortem specimens collected from dead eland, buffalo and kudu tissues from each of the National Parks and amplified by reverse transcription PCR using rinderpest fusion protein gene-specific primers (Forsyth and Barrett, 1995). Sequence analysis of the DNA product was carried out using standard DNA sequencing methods and phylogenetic comparisons with earlier virus isolates were carried out using the PHYLIP computer programme (Felsenstein, 1990). Based on an analysis of archived strains, rinderpest strains had already been classified into four distinct phylogenetic lineages.

One lineage is represented by the contemporary vaccine strain, derived from a field strain circulating in Kenya in 1911 and conserved in the laboratory ever since. As there are no more recent representatives of this lineage, it is assumed to have died out. The remaining rinderpest strains can be grouped into three contemporary lineages, one from Asia and two from Africa. The majority of recent African isolates belong to Africa lineage 1, which is currently present in an endemic area taking in southern Sudan and northern Uganda. In East Africa the historical strains RBT/1 (isolated in January 1961) and RGK/1 strain (isolated in January, 1962) had been shown to belong to lineage 2 but as no more recent isolate was available it was assumed that as far as East Africa was concerned, lineage 2 had also died out. At continental level, Africa lineage 2 virus was last isolated in Sokoto, in West Africa in 1983.

The consternation that now arose was due to the fact that the wildlife viruses from 1994, 5 & 6 all belonged to lineage 2. Barrett et al., (1998) point out that in spite of the high mutability of viral RNA, there are precedents for viruses within an ecological niche remaining relatively stable. This prompted the conclusion that the 1994-6 viruses were more than likely the direct descendants of the field strains circulating in East Africa in the early 60's. In other words rinderpest had been able undergo a remarkable adaptation and continue field transmission for 30 years without attracting veterinary attention.

6.3 The long-term persistence of cryptic rinderpest

The clue as to how this might have happened lay in a study of the virulence of one of the contemporary virus isolates. Even though the number of experimental animals was small, it was immediately apparent that it was producing a mild form of the disease in three of the four animals into which it was inoculated. Given that whilst mild in cattle the same virus is highly pathogenic for buffalo, eland and kudu, it seems that a virus similar in nature to that reported by Robson et al in 1959 was still in existence. In northern Tanzania in the early 60's, when the presence of mild strains was recognised but not the difficulty they would subsequently cause, it was accepted that Masai stock owners would only report clinical disease in times of drought. Thus it can be postulated that even while retaining a pathogenicity for game animals, in parts of East Africa where game animals were relatively sparse, and where their death might easily go unnoticed, mild rinderpest could easily persist over long periods of time through sub-clinical cattle to cattle transmission. As mild strains were known to be present in both Kenya and Tanzania in the early 60's, and as there was never any subsequent survey work to show that they had been eliminated, the postulate remains valid. Even if there had been an occasional flare up of clinical disease under adverse conditions, unless anticipated and diligently sought for, such incidents may well have passed without comment. As Plowright (1998) notes, there are plenty of other conditions in East Africa with which such low-grade mortality might have been confused.

6.4 Possible reversions to virulence

The spectre of infectious avirulent rinderpest presents regulators with a variety of problems. Not least of these will be their inability to produce serological evidence to show that a population within which such a virus is circulating is free of rinderpest, even if no disease is noted. As a result of this the country or zone will fail to gain OIE acceptance as being free from the virus and therefore any existing trade restrictions will remain in place. The other point is that conditions may develop under which there could be a reversion to virulence. It is perhaps worthwhile exploring two instances where this might have occurred although in neither case is conclusive evidence available.

In mid-1980, fourteen years after avirulent rinderpest was last clinically detected in Tanzania, abnormal mortalities were recorded in giraffe, eland and gazelles in Tanzanian villages close to the Kenyan border and to the Tsavo National Park. In the intervening period there had been no serological follow-up to determine that Tanzania was free from infection and latterly, budgetary restrictions had severely diminished the reporting capabilities of the national veterinary service. On investigation it was discovered that in Mwanga District an outbreak associated with mortality in cattle had been going on from May to July 1980. Although the initial diagnosis was confused with East Coast Fever (ECF), some animals were found with oral necrosis and *post mortem* examinations showed catarrhal and haemorrhagic gastroenteritis which, along with the diarrhoea, are signs more consistent with rinderpest (against which the animals would not have been vaccinated).

Throughout the remainder of 1980 and the whole of 1981, game animal species continued to die in a number of locations in northern Tanzania. Although still not confirmed as rinderpest it is possible to view these events as evidence of the disease creeping southwards and westwards from an outbreak that started as a focus on the Kenyan border in mid-1980. In March 1982 rinderpest was eventually recognised and confirmed in Lobo, in the north of the Serengeti National Park. By June that year it was recognised that there had been a substantial die-off of buffaloes in the Ngorongoro Conservation Authority Area where between 2000 & 4000 deaths were thought to have occurred (Rossiter *et al.*, 1983). Deaths in cattle were also reported from mid-1982 onwards in a contiguous area of northern Tanzania and the presence of rinderpest in the bovine population was confirmed serologically in 5 of 24 samples collected in November 1982 (Taylor & Nyange, unpublished results).

Local Masai pastoralists concluded by themselves that the disease was rinderpest, and non-pastoralists stated that it was the worst outbreak they had experienced for over 40 years. The main epidemiological issue however, the origin of the outbreak, remained unresolved. Sequence analysis was not available at this time and no virus was isolated. In the absence of an established connection between the events in northern Tanzania in 1980-82 and the lineage 1 endemic area in the south of Sudan, and in the absence of evidence showing that Tanzania was free of avirulent rinderpest infection, one possible explanation would be that the origins of the outbreak were internal and represented the recrudescence of virulence of the avirulent strain from a persistently cryptic focus, possibly associated with a build up of high excretion levels by passage in game animals. While no evidence can be placed in support of this hypothesis, the events of 1980-82 bear considerable resemblance to those of 1994-96 in southern Kenya except that in the latter instance a prompter diagnosis and responsiveness may have prevented the development greater virulence for cattle.

In Egypt, after two or three false starts, rinderpest established itself as an acutely endemic infection in 1903; it was regularly reported until 1927 and apparently continuously present up until 1967. There then ensued a period of 14 years (1967-1981) when the country was considered free of the disease. During that period when vaccine coverage was limited to a single campaign every two years for all bovines over two years of age. A fresh, apparently virulent epidemic commenced in 1982 and lasted until 1986. In 1984, in the course of this epidemic, a strain of rinderpest was isolated (Taylor, 1986) which was shown to be capable of causing silent infections in some experimental cattle, but moderately severe infection in others (E.Anderson, personal communication). It has always been difficult to link the origins of this epidemic with any known focus of a virulent form of the disease. So, once again, the possibility arises that an apathogenic strain of rinderpest could have circulated silently within the population for a number of years. This hypothesis would suggest that the apparently sudden onset of the epidemic might have been due to this virus regaining its virulence. To some extent the prior existence of such an apathogenic variant is borne out by the isolation of a virus with this character in 1984, while its ability to behave with a higher level of virulence in certain individual animals might indicate that it contained more than one virulence variant.

It is unfortunate that the bovine animal remains the only model system by which we can estimate the virulence of different rinderpest viruses; it is nevertheless still available to us. Under these circumstances it is possible to conclude that all the tools necessary for fully comprehending and monitoring the adaptiveness of rinderpest in the field are available. The fact that we have failed to do so in the past must not be allowed to happen in the future. It is therefore extremely important that every attempt is made to isolate field viruses whenever possible. Even though a number of the points discussed in the present section are not scientifically verified, within GREP it is important to try to understand how rinderpest has been able to go undetected for long periods of time and to learn how to rule out the same pattern repeating itself.

6.5 Is the virulence of PPR also variable?

In the Middle East we may be observing the ability of PPR to gain an endemic presence within a country without causing an initial heavy mortality in the resident small ruminant populations.

Although not well studied, it is possible that the virulence of this related morbillivirus is just as variable as that of rinderpest. Unlike rinderpest, with PPR there are few instances where lengthy vaccination campaigns have been directed at the control of this virus. Therefore, taking into account the outcome of some of the recent findings with rinderpest it may be argued that for both these viruses a low level of field virulence is the normal situation, and that high levels of virulence represent the aberrant situation. On this basis highly adapted low virulence strains may represent the basis on which a number of dangerously unobtrusive transboundary events take place. Such strains might later revert to a more virulent character. The possibility that these are field realities calls for the development of special surveillance routines with the capacity to detect transboundary incursions of strains of low virulence. These are seen as being immediately justified in countries bordering known rinderpest or PPR infected territories, even if for the time being the results demonstrate that no spread has occurred.

In India we have now seen evidence to show that PPR regularly infects in-contact bovines which undergo a silent, presumably non-transmissible, infection. There is also recent evidence to suggest that PPR may cause a clinical disease and death in the domestic buffalo (Govindrajan et al, 1997). It is still not clear if this was an isolated or a representative instance, either of which might indicate the possible adaptation to a new host from which virus transmission might be considered possible. Thus in a number of ways now is the correct time to begin to study of the virulence of morbilliviruses, how this may affect host range and transmission and how it may be, and is, modulated under field conditions. It may be noted that by sequencing the entire genome of a virulent and an attenuated variant of rinderpest, no progress could be made in furthering this understanding. Now, using DNA transcripts of the viruses, individual whole genes can be exchanged and work is currently in progress transposing them from virulent rinderpest into the attenuated virus; no results are yet available. It would seem that a similar initiative is needed to explore the virulence of PPR.

7. Seromonitoring

7.1 What is seromonitoring?

Seromonitoring is the application of an antibody determination technique to estimate the prevalence of immunised animals in a livestock population involved in a vaccination campaign. The technique of drawing up sampling frames, defining sampling units, the random selection of sampling units to be visited and of collecting and testing serum samples is well understood. Within the PARC programme, where there has been a heavy reliance on classic blanket vaccination campaigns to rid countries of rinderpest, National Campaign Co-ordinators (NCC's) have perceived the need to have a means of estimating the efficacy of the work output of their vaccination teams. Correctly generated this information can be used by NCC's to estimate the likelihood of rinderpest still persisting after completion of a particular vaccination campaign. In this they have been greatly assisted by the International Atomic Energy Agency which has ensured that the relevant ELISA technology was developed, standardised and transferred to a series of national laboratories throughout Africa. This endeavour has ensured that the output and progress of national vaccination campaigns is transparent both to local managers and to international sponsors.

As the purpose of seromonitoring is primarily to provide local managers with a tool for assessing the effectiveness of their vaccination campaigns it is essential that both the sampling skills and the laboratory skills should be available at national level before any vaccination campaign commences.

7.2 The dynamics of seromonitoring

In introducing rinderpest seromonitoring Tyler (1991) pointed out that for best management results the technique should be used as a dynamic tool to look at the effectiveness of individual campaigns undertaken in individual administrative regions within a country. Under these circumstances the important criterion was to measure the prevalence of herds with immunity levels sufficient to interrupt virus transmission. In sampling it was important to develop a sampling frame that included the entire livestock population undergoing vaccination and within this frame to randomly select village herds to be visited and sampled.

As a result of the occurrence of a number of outbreaks of rinderpest in northern Tanzania between 1982 & 1984 a series of donor funded blanket rinderpest vaccination campaigns were undertaken. The emergency situation having apparently been controlled by emergency vaccination campaigns, the objective of these campaigns was to create a belt of immunised animals throughout the whole of Tanzania. This activity was seen as providing a high level of security to livestock living in countries to the south of Tanzania; it was seen to be doing this by simultaneously providing additional assurance that the virus' transmission chain within Tanzania had been severed .and preventing the possible spread of infection from a more northerly neighbour to a southern one. As is so frequent in the design of such programmes, it was not entirely clear how, apart from vaccinating several million head of cattle, the probability that either of these objectives could be accomplished, was to be measured. In the event an attempt was made to reach and immunise all the cattle in each of the 82 Districts of the country through a programme of simultaneous vaccination in each of the country's 22 administrative regions. Even though the presence of an infected area had been established, it would probably be correct to say that had the national herd been uniformly immunised to a prevalence of 85%, even if only briefly maintained, then the continued persistence of rinderpest would have been unlikely. However, to provide a long-term guarantee that the whole of Tanzania was capable of acting as a vaccine buffer zone, it would have been necessary to maintain the same high level of immunity throughout the entire programme. The campaigns were undertaken between May and September in each of 1995, 1996 & 1997. Seromonitoring was undertaken.

In general samples with which to monitor post-campaign immunity levels were only collected at the time of the next campaign, i.e. nearly 12 months post vaccination. However, when cattle from selected districts were sampled within a month of vaccination and then again one year later, the results were as shown below.

Prevalence of rinderpest-immune cattle at an interval of 12 months in selected districts of Tanzania

District	% immune after one month	% immune after 12 months
Korogwe	31	32
Handeni	34	17
Moshi	64	18
Mwanga	45	44
Arusha	48	34
Mbulu	63	42
Kilombero	54	50
Mpwapwa	64	34
Nsasi	63	37

Looking at these results two things are immediately apparent. The first is that in most instances the prevalence of immune animals was unacceptably low immediately after completion of the vaccination campaign. Secondly, that in 2/3rds of the districts sampled the percentage of immune animals in the population waned over the following 12 months, in some cases by as much as 50%. Later, after the third round of annual vaccination, when the prevalence of immunity in individual age groups was examined, it was shown that three annual rounds were required before a particular cohort of animals developed a level of immunity approaching 85-90%. On the other hand cohorts of animals exposed to only one or two annual campaigns ended up with immunity levels substantially below this figure.

Even though satisfactory levels were attained in some instances, the final country-wide analysis showed mean immunity levels ranging from 48% in animals less than a year old to 76% in animals over 3 years old. It was apparent that in each age group there were wide variations in the prevalence rates both between and within districts.

These results provide an excellent illustration of the dynamic possibilities of seromonitoring as a tool for the production of data that should permit managers to assess the effectiveness of their campaigns. In this example although the seromonitoring managers had proposed the collection of samples one month after vaccination ended, they faced practical difficulties that made them adopt a different sampling scheme. Unfortunately, by routinely sampling many months after the individual campaigns had ended, the managers were unable to determine exactly how effective their vaccination work had actually been. From this study it became clear that the future of vaccination work lay in using it to undertake carefully defined and epidemiologically valid objectives, under a management equipped to implement immediate post-campaign seromonitoring from which results could be rapidly obtained. It was also necessary to foresee contingency facilities in order to instigate immediate revaccination where the first results are unsatisfactory. The success of any revaccination would then to be verified by further seromonitoring.

7.3 PARC Seromonitoring

Between 1991 and 1996 the rinderpest vaccination campaigns undertaken in West Africa under the aegis of the PARC have repeatedly demonstrated district and regional herd immunity levels below 85%. Unfortunately, this information has seldom been set against the decline in the number of recorded outbreaks (rinderpest is unknown in West Africa since 1988) in order to stimulate programme managers into asking if there is a point in constantly striving to reach an arbitrary target prevalence figure when it is distinctly probable that the virus had already been eradicated. The results obtained suggests that it may well have been possible to break the transmission chain either by locally efficient vaccination campaigns or by inefficient ones supplemented by non-specific factors. In the field disease control procedures may improve across the board when the vaccination teams are working alongside the livestock community and communicating with livestock owners on a daily basis. Unfortunately, in a number of instances seromonitoring results have been evaluated to indicate a need for further attempts to raise the percentage of immunity in the national herds even though the no recent outbreaks have been recorded. As a result it has often been unclear whether campaign managers are still intent on eradicating the virus or whether their strategy has changed to that of fortifying the national herd against the re-entry of the virus from an external source. In either case it is unlikely that continued vaccination is serving any real end.

7.4 Seromonitoring in South Asia

In India the need for seromonitoring was slow to be appreciated. As a consequence no seromonitoring was undertaken before putting an end to the mass vaccination programme against rinderpest that had been going on for a number of years throughout northern India - and declaring that part of the sub-continent provisionally rinderpest-free. In fact the absence of seromonitoring results may have made it easier to end vaccination when it did as, had seromonitoring results been available they might have been so unsatisfactory that national mangers might have found it more difficult than they already did to persuade locally responsible officers to make such an apparently dangerous decision based only on the absence of recorded disease outbreaks. Subsequently when vaccination work was concentrated within what appeared to be the last infected area in southern India, seromonitoring results indicated that if, as seemed to be the case, the transmission chain had been broken, it had done so with immunity levels considerably lower than 85%; again the role of non-specific factors may have played a part.

7.5 Seromonitoring is most effective immediately the campaign is complete

During the course of a transboundary rinderpest incursion in Tanzania in 1997 considerable emphasis was placed on delineating the infected area. Subsequently it was decided to vaccinate the cattle population within this area in order to break any onward transmission of the virus. Seromonitoring was undertaken and the results processed on completion of the initial vaccination work. The results indicated that from the prevalence of immunity detected the required outcome could not be guaranteed. Accordingly a second round of vaccination was immediately undertaken in the same population followed, also immediately by a second round of seromonitoring. In each instance the need for seromonitoring was foreseen, budgeted and completed within a few weeks of the end of the actual vaccination work. The final seromonitoring results obtained (see below) supported the conclusion that rinderpest ought to have been eradicated and that it would be a waste of resources to continue with further campaigns.

Rinderpest antibody prevalences after the first and second phases of emergency vaccination

District	Rinderpest antibody % prevalence range		Mean % prevalence		No villages with prevalence of >85%	
	First phase	Second phase	First phase	Second phase	First phase	Second phase
Ngorongoro	33.3-95%	75-100	75	87.0	4/24	23/24
Monduli	16-91.7%	33.3-100	65.5	94.4	2/24	17/24

7.6 Problems associated with assessing the results of seromonitoring

Experience has shown that the technology with which to undertake seromonitoring has been successfully transferred and maintained in a number of LDCs. Frequently however, this has only served to demonstrate the absence of a care in determining the original objectives of mounting the vaccination campaign and how monitoring might demonstrate whether or not these had been achieved. As a result the successful transfer of an appropriate technology has left international co-ordinators unaware of the need to provide training and advice on how to obtain focused seromonitoring results, how to assess them and how to adapt strategic plans on the basis of the outcome.

8. Serosurveillance

8.1 The value of serosurveillance

Serosurveillance is the technique applied to the detection of antibodies arising as a result of natural infection as opposed to vaccination. While the technique for estimating the presence of antibodies may well be the same as that used in seromonitoring, the reason for looking for them within a population is quite different. With the serosurveillance approach, a positive antibody detection implies that the animal from which the sample was drawn has experienced infection with the agent in question. A negative result implies that the animal has not experienced the infection. Serosurveillance is therefore a technique that can be used to determine whether or not an infectious agent is, or has been present within a population. With the correct choice of the age group of animals sampled it should also be possible to determine whether this information is contemporary or historic. This offers two practical applications of the technique. In the first place by detecting specific antibodies in young animals, it can be used either to indicate the presence of infection in different sub-populations and therefore, when sufficient sub-populations have been examined, to reveal the distribution of the infection within the population as a whole. It can also be used in the same manner to generate evidence that the agent in question is no longer replicating in the population being examined.

Unfortunately, in most cases it is difficult to distinguish between the immune response to vaccine and that to field infection. Therefore serosurveillance is not normally practicable in populations undergoing vaccination.

As the purpose of serosurveillance is primarily epidemiological requiring managerial ability in defining the purpose of the investigation, in determining where, how many and what sort of samples should be collected (and recollected if necessary) and in evaluating the meaning of the results. In parallel, laboratory technology, resources and skills must also be available to process the samples. Therefore within any control or eradication programme, in order to link programme management to epidemiological results it is essential that all aspects of the serosurveillance technique be available at national level.

8.2 The importance of ageing the animals sampled

While the serological tests are often relatively simple to perform, a sample of an animal population which includes animals of all ages usually discloses only that some animals have antibodies to the disease in question. From such an observation it would only be possible to conclude that the population had experienced infection at some time in the past, but the remoteness of that experience could not be determined. However, this information can be given considerably more meaning with a knowledge of the ages of the animals from which the samples were taken which should facilitate the distinction between a previous or a contemporary infection. If animals of all age groups are sampled it may be possible to see, if the infection has ended, when it ended. With rinderpest one of the earliest examples of the use of serosurveillance was the work of Taylor & Watson (1967), investigating the possible maintenance of rinderpest in the various wildebeest populations of the Serengeti National Park in northern Tanzania. Samples were collected from animals provisionally aged by the spread of the horns and verified by an examination of dentition and the number of scars left by the corpora lutea of pregnancy (assuming regular annual conceptions). Using these techniques it was possible assemble a collection of serum samples representing all age groups within the community. Using a virus neutralisation test the results showed that rinderpest infected these animals in the years up to 1961 but not in any of the years thereafter. Although numerous animals born to different older age groups carried antibodies to the virus (i.e. they were seropositive) it was impossible to conclude whether or not they were infected during their first year of life, or whether a single episode accounted for the development of antibodies in animals of a number of different age groups. On the other hand it was clear that the populations being sampled had been free of infection for 4 to 5 years and were not maintaining the virus.

8.3 The role of serosurveillance in determining freedom from infection

In view of the possible development of an avirulent strain of rinderpest in a population undergoing vaccination, the Office International des Epizooties (OIE) decided that it would not accept the absence of clinically reported rinderpest as evidence that a population was totally free of the virus. Rather, it foresaw a requirement for serosurveillance results as a means of proving that there was no cryptic virus circulating within the population. Unfortunately a number.of the populations to which serosurveillance is currently applicable have a history of the use of rinderpest vaccine in their earlier fight against the clinical disease. Up to the present time rinderpest vaccines do not carry a marker which will allow laboratories to distinguish between post-vaccinal and post-infection rinderpest antibodies. Therefore, meaningful serosurveillance can only be undertaken in a population of unvaccinated animals. To underline this point the OIE now requires an undertaking that any country wishing to have its apparent rinderpest-free status internationally accepted has to cease rinderpest vaccination. This it does when it makes its declaration of provisional freedom from rinderpest. If it enjoys a further three years without the reappearance of the clinical disease, it may apply for disease-free recognition. This status however, is not the equivalent of recognition as infection-free.

Recognition of the latter status must also be applied for but, in order to make such an application, it is vital to have serological data which can be interpreted as demonstrating the absence of persistence of the virus within the population. The conditions that govern the various stages in the certification of a country as rinderpest infection-free are described as the (so called) OIE Pathway (OIE, 1998). This states that serosurveillance of a previously vaccinated population should not begin until at least two years after the date vaccination ended, this being the time deemed necessary to accrue a meaningful population of potentially susceptible cattle in which to undertake the surveillance work. If this population is kept under serological observation for two consecutive years thereafter, with no evidence of unvaccinated animals developing rinderpest antibodies, then there are epidemiological grounds for concluding that wild virus is absent as a result of which an infection-free status may be granted.

8.4 Difficulties in the interpretation of serosurveillance results

As a group the north-east states of India declared themselves provisionally free of rinderpest in 1994 and commenced to install serosurveillance technology in 1995, including field serum collection and testing with the competition ELISA test (OIE, 1996). In view of the fact that some vaccination work had been undertaken in the years before 1994 it was possible that rinderpest antibodies might be detected in animals younger than one year old or in animals more than 24 months of age. Although not so far demonstrated in South Asia, the presence of avirulent field strains of rinderpest in that region remains a theoretical possibility. The more so in the light of the observations of Littlewood (1905) that cattle from Asia Minor would often be affected with rinderpest without showing any clinical symptoms, particularly during the summer. It is therefore extremely important to rule out this possibility. In the first attempts to do this, one state demonstrated the presence of rinderpest antibodies in 12-18 month old animals in a group of adjacent villages, evidence consistent with the presence of such a virus. The appearance of this evidence caused considerable consternation which had to be resolved through a fact-finding mission. Fortunately, when such a mission was undertaken, it was found that a zealous local veterinarian had discovered some old rinderpest vaccine in his store and decided to use it in a local campaign, even though a directive against such campaigns had been issued one year earlier. When the same villages were retested a year later there was no evidence of further seroconversion (when the serological profile of an infected animal turns from negative to positive). This experience pointed out firstly how hard it was to ensure that local officials in remote areas totally are immediately compliant with central instructions and how such instructions should have included the surrender of any unused rinderpest vaccine. It also demonstrated the danger of a hasty interpretation of serosurveillance results and how, unless accompanied by improved training at all levels, major serosurveillance schemes may be beset by problems in interpreting their results. They also demonstrated that even if the underlying laboratory system is working correctly, serosurveillance is not a technique that can suddenly be introduced and expected to provide unequivocal results as soon as it is introduced. In situations where the outcome will impact on a nation's trading interests, it is vital that the introduction of serosurveillance is accompanied by a technically and epidemiologically competent trouble-shooting support teams.

In looking at serosurveillance results it is important to remember that immunoglobulins are transferred through colostrum and that young animals may possess a maternal immunity which cannot readily be distinguished from an active one. It is therefore important to determine exactly when maternal immunity is likely to wane to an undetectable level. With rinderpest there has been an element of confusion over this point although the work of Brown (1958) showed that the time to the disappearance of maternal antibodies was highly variable but that the mean extinction point was 9 months +/- 2 months. These results showed that in some animals maternal antibodies might be present until the recipient was 11 months old.

In Egypt there has been no apparent clinical disease since 1986 but nevertheless, based on previous experience, there is an awareness that subclinical rinderpest may still be present. At the same time it has been considered necessary to maintain vaccination coverage until this point was resolved, presenting technicians with the problem of undertaking serosurveillance in a highly immune population. Since April 1993 this has been attempted using sera collected from unvaccinated cattle and buffalo calves over 8 months of age in the belief that these should be maternal antibody free. The results have shown that 10% of the cattle sampled (118/11191) are rinderpest antibody positive, as are 20.4% (102/501) of buffaloes. These antibodies have been rationalised in terms of i) mixed-up samples, ii) persistent passive immunity iii) the calves having been vaccinated or iv) circulating virus. In looking at this explanation the point to be appreciated is that after eliminating administrative problems, because animals that might still be demonstrating maternal immunity were being tested, it was impossible to distinguish between that possibility, and that of a circulating virus. Again a problem was being encountered that could be attributed to a lack of skills in the management of serosurveillance. To resolve the issue, all that was necessary was to adjust the sampling age of the animals to between 12 and 12 to 15/18 months.

8.5 Managing serosurveillance

In spite of being an extremely powerful epidemiological tool serosurveillance the intricacies of planning surveys that will yield unequivocal results is not a well developed skill. The ELISA test has been transferred to laboratories in developing countries far more successfully than the epidemiologists skills with which to undertake good surveys. Serosurveillance is now virtually the only tool which will reveal the extent of the rinderpest-infected area within East Africa but evidence that management can envisage how it is to be utilised to that end is still awaited. Equally, in India there is now a pressing need to use serosurveillance to demonstrate the presence or absence of cryptic rinderpest in the largely unvaccinated bovine population throughout the sub-continent. It is now vital to demonstrate that resources can be responsibly managed to obtain a speedy resolution of both these serosurveillance issues.

9. Techniques for controlling infectious diseases

9.1 Methods

Infectious diseases maintain themselves in nature through an endless chain of transmission events in which an infected individual acts as a donor and a susceptible individual, usually within the same community, acts as a recipient. There are essentially only two ways in which this chain can be broken. One of these involves taking steps which will prevent the donor fulfilling its role. The other involves the use of immunisation of susceptible hosts to curtail their role as recipients of infection. These general principles apply in the fields of human and veterinary medicine alike.

10. Breaking the transmission chain without vaccines

10.1 The use of isolation facilities

In a small community preventing contact between an infectious donor and susceptible members of that community can be achieved in a number of ways. In human medicine infectious individuals used to be sequestrated in so called isolation hospitals, outside the main body of the community. In veterinary medicine temporary housing might be erected in order to isolate infected cattle outside a village (Littlewood, 1905). The creation of a physical distance between the infectious donor and potential recipients of that donor's infection was generally effective in creating a barrier across which the agent could not spread. In human medicine however, such a situation posed considerable risks for medical and nursing staff alike and newer and safer ways of sequestering infectious patients were sought. Barrier nursing was the result. With the emergence of a variety of highly pathogenic organisms such as Ebola and Lassa fever viruses such measures were essential.

10.2 The continuing relevance of stamping out measures in veterinary medicine

In veterinary medicine somewhat different solutions are generally sought. With highly infectious diseases such as Foot and Mouth Disease (FMD) where transmission is readily achieved by direct, and indirect contact as well as by aerosol dispersal, it has been accepted policy in a number of countries to slaughter the infected donors the moment they are identified. This is done in order to halt any further generation of any transmissible virus. To reduce the possibility of accidental transmission from the carcasses to susceptible hosts, the remains of the infected animals are disposed of by incineration or burial and the premises are thoroughly disinfected. Clearly such measures are unpopular within the farming community as farming is about profitability, and so they must have a strong legal backing and enforcement procedures. Essentially this means that veterinary services must be prepared to prosecute defaulters and exact all the penalties prescribed by law. On the other hand, the farming community may well expect compensation for the loss of animals slaughtered for the public good and this should obviously be forthcoming.

10.3 Alternative solutions for use in communities sensitive to the destruction of livestock and the requirement for legal powers

In the case of less infectious diseases stamping out procedures may be modified. Salem Bey (1947) showed that rinderpest did not transmit when donor and susceptible recipients were separated by an air space one metre in width. This led Taylor and Nanda (1995) to propose household or farm sequestration, instead of slaughter, as a policy for breaking the rinderpest infection chain in India. Even though less severe than slaughter, a sequestration policy still requires that the concerned Veterinary Authorities be given powers compelling livestock owners to notify the presence of animals that could be suffering from rinderpest or any other infectious disease, powers to enter farms and farm buildings in order to examine animals and collect samples, and powers to declare a farm an infected premises. Additional powers must be available which will enable the Veterinary Authorities to bar the movement of animals from the infected premises until recovered (i.e. sequester them on the premises) and to compel the owner, his family and his staff from coming in contact with livestock on other farms within the village. It must also be possible to declare the area surrounding the village to be a restricted area within which the movement of livestock is prohibited except by special licence (e.g. animals for immediate slaughter, vacation of premises adjoining the infected one etc.) and within which no public marketing of livestock is permitted. While sympathetic to the concept that compulsory slaughter will alienate the community it may nevertheless remain a desirable option and funds should be available to compensate an owner voluntarily permitting the slaughter of his infected stock. Powers should also be available to compel the sanitary disposal of animals that succumb to the disease. Finally if the application of the above measures is failing to control the disease situation and national livestock security is being compromised, emergency powers of compulsory slaughter should nevertheless be available. Finally, powers should be available to compel the disinfection of selected premises and vehicles.

10.4 Difficulties with quarantines

In situations where nomadism, transhumance or trekking trade animals are integral to the life style of stock owners, sequestration generally gives way to measures aimed at quarantining a group of infected animals to prevent them transmitting the disease to other livestock communities. Unfortunately, although the veterinary authorities may have the legal powers to apply these measures, they are seldom given sufficient support by the civil administration to make them effective. In part this may be attributed to the logistics of enforcing such an exercise as the owner will not accept a quarantine situation in which he is unable to ensure adequate fodder and water for his stock. Probably of greater importance is the deteriorating value of slaughter stock which tempts the owner to break the quarantine and attempt to introduce his animals infected into the market. In the African rinderpest epidemic of the early 80s it was not uncommon to hear accounts of ailing trek animals being moved to markets in central Africa on vehicles before their value deteriorated. During the same episode, when a newly introduced rinderpest-infected herd escaped from quarantine in eastern Nigeria, the livestock losses caused by the subsequent spread of rinderpest throughout that country caused severe economic hardship (Nawathe & Lamorde, 1984).

On the other hand is likely that a pro-sequestration policy contributed to the rapid elimination of rinderpest from India in the years between 1990 and 1995. At the very least its open discussion may have discouraged the illegal movement and marketing of infected animals which had probably contributed to the sporadic incidence of rinderpest in the urban dairies of northern India in the previous decade. In view of the immense unpopularity of a mandatory slaughter policy on the sub-continent what is now needed is a means of adapting the same policy to the more highly infectious diseases such as FMD. Obviously it would not be possible to sequester FMD -infected animals in individual households but it would be possible to impound village animals in large enclosures until they had recovered from the infection. However, the infectious secretions such animals would generate might easily carry the virus to a neighbouring village and it would therefore be important to prevent this happening. This might be achieved by placing the stock in large portable barns inflated by compressed air and maintained under negative internal pressure and with HEPA filtration being applied to the exhaust air and strict controls applied to the movement of handlers and the safe disposal of waste materials.

11 Breaking the transmission chain with vaccines and vaccination campaigns

11.1 The immunisation policy

The use of vaccine to immunise otherwise susceptible hosts is an alternative way of interrupting the transmission chain. So effective is this strategy that it is almost invariably seen as the only solution available in the fight against infectious diseases.

Usually a vaccination policy is introduced either in the knowledge that it will not be immediately possible to immunise the entire at-risk population or if it is, that the risk of the re-introduction of infection from neighbouring populations will mean that the policy must be pursued indefinitely. Frequently vaccination will be introduced in an endemic disease situation as a means of ensuring the survival of the most highly valued genetic material within a country. After this there will generally be a lengthy period during which, although the effects of the agent may be diminished, it will probably continue to circulate within the population. Ultimately it may be possible for a group of countries in a similar phase of advanced disease control to apply the same vaccination policy in a drive towards eradication. However, in accepting vaccination as a national control policy for a particular disease causing agent there should be a broad level of understanding between the public animal health authorities and the livestock industry as to the likely costs involved. The crucial issue of course is related to who should pay for the on-going interventions, the industry or the taxpayer. While of these issues can usually be resolved one way or the other within the strong world economies, their solution is far more problematic in the LDCs.

11.2 The introduction of vaccine strategies

Unfortunately, in many poorly performing countries, the foundations of the livestock industry are threatened by a bewildering array of pathogenic organisms against which the individual farmer is virtually powerless to act. Inevitably, attempting to underpin the security of this industry is seen as a public good, and national veterinary services were called upon to provide a free service to the best of their ability. Thus for many years the veterinary services of west and east Africa struggled to reduce the impact of rinderpest using herd quarantine policies, treatment with hyperimmune serum or protection with an inactivated vaccine which was difficult to distribute and only available in limited quantities. There was no question of the owner contributing to the costs and the objective was a mixture of acceptance of a civic responsibility to stop the virus spreading to an uninfected neighbour as to securing the basis for economic progress at the domestic level.

It was only around 1940 that the first generation of cheap, live attenuated vaccine became available that policy changes became apparent. In the first instance the new vaccine was used in much the same manner as before, in attempting to quench infection in an infected herd and to ring immunise animals possibly in contact with this herd. In East Africa it was not until epidemiological observations indicated that wildlife species were aiding the distribution of the virus that this policy was finally discarded. In its place a new policy was instigated in an attempt to interrupt the transmission chain by vaccinating all the susceptible bovines throughout the infected region of the country (Branagan & Hammond, 1965). This change to a mass vaccination policy could not have been contemplated without the availability of the attenuated vaccine; it also carried with it the hope that in the short term eradication would follow its introduction. Throughout the process of reviewing and evolving more and more appropriate strategies rinderpest control remained a public sector undertaking. The fact that nearly 50 years later, eradication attempts are still being made and that the process is more expensive, complicated and difficult than ever before, suggests that something went wrong in between.

11.3 From attenuated rinderpest vaccines to failed eradication schemes

The development of different generations of attenuated rinderpest vaccines came about as a result of a publicly funded research programmes looking for new and more effective ways to combat the disease. Both the first and second generation attenuated rinderpest vaccines were shown to be highly efficacious and were generally considered to provide life-long immunity if given to a fully susceptible hosts (Plowright & Taylor, 1967). Although initially used to protect selected highly valuable stock once that objective has been achieved their use become more and more widespread and undoubtedly succeeded in reducing the general weight of rinderpest infection. By persisting with national rinderpest control policies, a number of countries were very successful. For instance through the use of rinderpest vaccine Kenya, Uganda and Tanzania apparently all but eliminated the infection in the years between 1961 and 1967 (Atang & Plowright, 1969). At the same time, because of its very success in controlling rinderpest, the vaccination policy required could not be abandoned even though the amount of vaccine required, and the cost of producing and administering it, were constantly increasing. Obviously the only effective solution to this recurrent cycle would be to increase the uptake of vaccine to the point where the virus' transmission chain was irrevocably broken and eradication achieved. Moreover, to stand any chance of making this solution permanent, it would be necessary to undertake the same programme at the same time within all parts of the infected area, even if that involved a number of neighbouring countries.

In both Africa and Asia such programmes were attempted. In India a National Rinderpest Eradication Programme was launched in 1956 with the epidemiologically valid objective of vaccinating 80% of the entire national bovine population in as short a time as possible. Follow-up campaigns were foreseen as being necessary to include annual herd recruits within this highly immune population. While correctly identifying the need for a rapid application of vaccine throughout all sectors of a population as a key principle in the total and simultaneous removal of all susceptible animals, they were unfortunate in not having the resources to match their implementation achievements to their ambitions. As a result in some states it was taking up to eight years to match vaccine uptake figures to the estimated bovine population. Not surprisingly rinderpest remained well entrenched for the next 30 years and the cost involved in maintaining whatever degree of control over the virus that had been achieved became a matter of national concern.

In Africa the Commission for Technical Co-operation in Africa South of the Sahara proposed a series of mass vaccination campaigns as a means of eradicating rinderpest. The resulting campaigns (collectively known as Joint Project 15 or JP15) were planned, organised and managed a in a series of phases, each involving the blanket annual vaccination of all cattle for three successive years. The first phase of the campaign started in the countries bordering Lake Chad in Central Africa in 1961 while the fourth phase and ended in Senegal in 1969. The campaigns were then switched to eastern Africa. A considerable part of the funding for JP15 was provided by external donors. At a technical level the project and its campaigns were a great success Although not subjected to routine seromonitoring, because 70% of the total annual vaccination work was discharged within a period of four months it is likely that a high proportion of the national herds involved were immunised at the same time. At the international level JP15 made no research provision and failed to see the need for long-term monitoring of the residual situation on the ground. Or contingency mechanisms (other than the efforts of the concerned national veterinary services) to deal with residual foci.

11.4 Continuing eradication programmes

In the 1980's India was still able to maintain control over
rinderpest but could not eradicate it. At the same time an internal review indicated that the disease seemed to be more entrenched in some parts of the country than in others. In 1990 India introduced a successful technical collaboration with the European Union for the time-bound eradication of rinderpest. Within this programme a group of programme managers had to propose a series of annual strategies and convince the implementing directorates at state-level of the correctness of their policies. In the event the last outbreak of Indian rinderpest was reported in 1995. In many respects the most important lesson that was learnt from this programme was the need to define the infected area, and concentrate appropriate resources within that area.

In Africa the situation developed less favourably as post JP15 residual foci did in fact exist and in the early 80s rinderpest was re-distributed over much of the terrain it had occupied before the start of the joint project. However, the difference was that now the concerned veterinary services no longer had the capacity, either physical or financial, to deal with the problem. External assistance was needed and this assistance would only be made available to countries prepared to critically examine a number of the problems they faced. In the event the Pan African Rinderpest Campaign (PARC) programme, which draws heavily on external funding from the European Union, has been instrumental both in designing ways of realigning the financing of national veterinary services and of eradicating rinderpest from West Africa; it has yet to repeat this success story in East Africa.

11.5 Interrupting rinderpest transmission through vaccination

Looking at the rinderpest model proposed by Rossiter & James (1989) it appears that if reliance is placed on herd immunity alone to interrupt the rinderpest transmission chain, then levels of around 85% will be required. On this basis it may be argued that a level below 85% might permit the continued circulation of the virus and simultaneously provide a selection pressure favouring the emergence of less virulent variants of the virus. Insights into national herd immunity levels in the pre-JP15 period were rarely possible and perhaps the best available data is that presented by Plowright to the Diamond Jubilee and Scientific Conference at Vom, Nigeria in 1984 in relation to Tanzania. In that country for many years the practice had been to vaccinate calves between 1 & 9 months of age and then to revaccinate them at between 13 & 21 months of age. In theory such animals would be immune for life and they were therefore branded after their second vaccination to indicate their rinderpest immune status. In two Provinces of Tanzania it was found that, by and large, branded animals had immunity rates of between 80 and 92%, younger unbranded animals might come from groups with immunity levels as low as 51%. In other words this policy, which had demonstrably eliminated clinical rinderpest from northern Tanzania, did not guarantee interruption of the chain of infection. Further, as has been argued above, it is possible that the persistence of an avirulent strain of rinderpest, the existence of which had already been demonstrated in Tanzania, might have been assisted by this policy.

On the other hand the very high levels of immunity Plowright was able to demonstrate in all age strata following a well organised JP15 pulsed vaccination campaign provides us with evidence that such campaigns should succeed in breaking the transmission chain and therefore in eradicating the virus. In the limited seromonitoring that accompanied JP15 in West Africa it was shown that after one pulse the herd overall herd immunity levels rose to around 70%, after a second pulse a year later it was around 90% but after a third pulse no substantial improvement could be achieved. Concomitantly the number of rinderpest outbreaks declined dramatically but not to zero. Therefore, on the much broader international scale, JP15 in fact demonstrated the same result. Even so, because of transhumant movements and the loss of maternal immunity, there was bound to be some waning of herd immunity levels in the period between annual successive campaigns. Taken together with the logistic impossibility of undertaking campaigns throughout the whole of West Africa simultaneously, some post-campaign foci of rinderpest had been anticipated. However, it was expected that zoosanitary policies would be used to stamp these out and the later reappearance of rinderpest in several countries suggests that these measures were not vigorously pursued. Nevertheless the success of JP15 clearly established the pulsed vaccination technique as a highly effective tool for interrupting the rinderpest transmission chain. Perhaps then the only drawback to such campaigns was that they fostered a feeling that vaccine technology itself guaranteed success and that more prosaic zoosanitary measures are of limited importance. This however, is not the case.

11.6 Does vaccination select a more adapted virus?

It has been said that vaccine is a virus' best friend. Looking at the emergence of avirulent rinderpest strains as a emerging contemporary problem, it is also possible that the two or three decades of partial vaccination of national herds before the start of JP15 provided a selection pressure that began a process of viral adaptation that has culminated in the development of a transmissible but attenuated strain of the virus. Once this process had begun, it is possible that such a virus could have escaped all but the most carefully organised vaccination campaigns. It has also been established that by the time JP15 transferred its activities from West to East Africa, such viruses had already evolved. It is also not disputed that JP15 was not as rigorously pursued in East Africa as in West Africa.

11.7 Vaccination is still a useful tool for eradicating viruses

We have recently developed a revised method of administering pulsed rinderpest vaccine in an area known to be infected with the avirulent rinderpest variant. In so doing the objective was declared to be the necessity of raising the prevalence rate of rinderpest immune bovines in the target population to over 85%. Accordingly, a crucial facet of this experiment was to estimate the prevalence of immunity immediately after the vaccination campaign ended, and this was done. As in the JP15 campaigns we were able to show that, although occasional herds developed high immunity levels in the population as a whole, a single round of vaccination achieved a prevalence of immunity of 70%. When this result became available it was immediately decided to revaccinate the entire target population in the hope of vaccinating 70% of the animals that were not presented at the first round. When the prevalence of immunity was re-estimated after the second round, it was now found to be just over 90%. On the basis of this result the population is being monitored clinically and serologically to ensure that no further virus transmission is occurring.

It is highly likely that vaccine will continue to find a ready application in eliminating rinderpest from the few areas where it remains a problem. In so doing it is important to avoid developing a situation that will make its clinical detection harder than it already is. It is therefore important to ensure that where vaccine is used, the campaigns are organised so as to achieve a high level of population immunity simultaneously throughout the whole of the target population. This requires careful logistical planning, the rapid administration of the vaccine and rapid post-campaign evaluation. It also requires a contingency plan for an immediate repetition of the campaign if the prevalence of immunity is below the desired figure.

11.8 A limited scope for bioengineered vaccines

There have been a number of attempts to develop bioengineered vaccines against rinderpest and while their efficacy is not questioned, the fact that rinderpest will probably be eradicated without using them suggests that there was no imperative reason why they should be developed. The existing tissue culture vaccine was deemed to be relatively thermolabile at high ambient temperatures, although its stability within a cold chain was not in doubt. Although recombinant rinderpest vaccines were seen as a means of ensuring an improved thermostability, introducing them in the middle of on-going eradication programmes risked throwing vaccine manufacturing procedures into turmoil. Instead, to overcome the thermostability problem Mariner et al, (1990) used an improved freeze drying protocol to develop a variant vaccine in which the dried virus was more slowly degraded than in the classic preparation. This thermostable rinderpest vaccine has been adopted in the field in areas of civil insecurity where veterinary cold chains do not exist Elsewhere, the availability of cold chains and a price differential have ensured the continuing popularity of the classic vaccine.

When bioengineered vaccines were in the early developmental stages it was considered important that they should be able to induce a duration of immunity comparable to that of the live attenuated vaccine. Now that rinderpest eradication is the goal rather than rinderpest control, the important issue is whether or not a population has been saturated with vaccine in a short space of time and the transmission chain broken; once this has been achieved, how long immunity lasts in individual animals is of lesser importance.

With the increasing need for serosurveillance to detect the presence of avirulent rinderpest strains, it is probably difficult to assure situations in which such surveillance work will always take place in unvaccinated populations. It would therefore be extremely useful if a contemporary manufacturer could incorporate an immunogenic marker protein into the existing vaccine in order to be able to use discriminatory ELISA tests to differentiate an antibody response to rinderpest vaccine from one to wild virus. A similar argument has been advanced for the use of a marked vaccine within rinderpest vaccine buffer zones, a point of some importance if the animal which had tested as serologically positive had moved outside the limits of the buffer zone. However, in countries that have eradicated rinderpest and wish to have this fact officially recognised, current thinking is that where there is a danger of re-infection from a contaminated neighbour, buffer zones are unlikely to be effective and should be replaced by zones in which active disease surveillance activities are given a high level of priority.

11.9 Fortress vaccination policies

In an attempt to buffer themselves against the possibility of re-infection with rinderpest from an external source, a number of West African countries appear to have adopted a policy of attempting to maintain a sufficiently high prevalence of immunity that an invading strain of the virus would be unable to establish itself. However, to indefinitely maintain a national herd immunity rate of over 85% must be viewed as virtually impossible. Moreover, under these circumstances it might be difficult to find clinical evidence of a virus incursion, even if the invading strain were moderately virulent, and very difficult if the strain were avirulent. Finally, the policy is impossible to defend from an economic point of view. A much more relevant policy would be one combining surveillance, both clinical and serological, with improved disease reporting and contingency planning.

11.10 The need for continuing research

Recent seromonitoring results from India showed that given vaccination teams working with given batches of rinderpest vaccine might expect highly variable rates of immunisation but the underlying reasons for this variability were not adequately investigated. Now, work in Saudi Arabia has shed light on a possible explanation for this well known problem. By recalling vials of vaccine which had been stored in the field it was possible to show that within a given batch the contents of some vials had deteriorated very rapidly where as others had retained the titre they were issued with. Thus if cattle in adjoining villages were vaccinated with the contents of a normal and a deteriorated vial, one village might have good results and the other appalling ones. In addition, it was shown that the post-reconstitution degradation rates might be considerably higher than those previously established. These observations illustrate the need for continual monitoring of the results of any vaccination campaign and the need to understand that with the passage of time, problems may occur in attempting to manufacture any standardised product. There is therefore a constant need to undertake applied research into keeping quality, degradation rates, the effects of breaks in the cold chain and into variable immunisation rates.

11.11 Is there a risk of PPR epidemics when rinderpest vaccination ends?

It is unfortunate that in India, as rinderpest has been eradicated, PPR has apparently spread to hitherto uninfected parts of the country while the level of outbreaks has reached epidemic proportions in those where it already occurred. Of course this apparent replacement of one morbillivirus by another may be entirely coincidental and no more than the outcome of improvements to disease surveillance and differential diagnosis. On the other hand it might be due to the selection of a more virulent PPR variant after release from a competitive selection pressure of which we have never been properly aware. In India for instance it can be suggested that PPR has existed there for many years but that its transmission rate was constantly modified by the inclusion of small ruminants in rinderpest vaccination programmes where they would develop a cross immunity to PPR. Under these circumstances it is possible that PPR adapted its transmission rate to survive within a partially immune population. When this selection pressure was removed by the eradication of rinderpest and the end of rinderpest vaccination in the small ruminant population, the virus may have developed a more aggressive variant which is currently spreading within the large, newly susceptible small ruminant population. In some states of southern India such a strain has been present for four years and through two major epidemic cycles without apparently showing any evidence of losing its virulence.

11.12 What vaccination policies are appropriate for controlling PPR

It is unlikely that many of the counties currently affected by PPR will attempt to eradicate the virus in the near future. They will therefore be left with little choice but to adopt vaccination policies aimed at achieving a level of control over the incidence of the virulent form of the disease. Probably the more economically viable sections of the livestock industry should be required to look after their own needs in this respect while limited public funds might be used to assist marginalised community members. Although conjectural, it is in fact possible to argue in support of a routine vaccination policy on the basis that, even if it selects for of a low-virulence variant, such a virus may well emerge in any situation involving long-term endemicity. In any event a programme should be set up to routinely monitor the virulence of field isolates of PPR using a standard assay system. With or without vaccination programmes, PPR virus should be subject to frequent isolations and its virulence assessed in order that any fluctuations are observed and documented.

Even if PPR with a low level of virulence is present in a country, strains may intermittently regain a higher level of virulence and so clinical outbreaks and associated mortality will probably continue to occur. If for any reason large susceptible populations have accrued, these may be severely involved. In seeking to prevent such occurrences through the constant use of vaccine a country puts itself livestock in the same situation that was characteristic of rinderpest infected countries before eradication campaigns were commenced. Under the circumstances in question there were sufficient resources to permit the use of vaccine to lower down the incidence of infection but insufficient resources to undertake eradication. Unfortunately, not able to move forwards, it was equally unacceptable to lessen control of the virus and in consequence a substantial proportion of the recurrent budget went into maintaining the status quo. Under such circumstances it finally became necessary to attract external donor funding in order to complete the task. Therefore, in moving towards the use of vaccine to control PPR it is important that Veterinary Services ensure that to a large extent the funding to sustain such a programme is met by those sections of the industry that can afford to make a contribution.

In theory PPR should be just as vulnerable to pulsed vaccination campaigns as rinderpest and therefore maintaining a high level of immunity in a rapidly regenerating small ruminant livestock population need not be the key to eradication that it is often seen to be. Rather, a single or multiple pulse of vaccination should quickly achieve the desired objective. However, as has been repeatedly demonstrated, eradication campaigns fail unless neighbouring countries work in concert with one another. Further, for there to be the necessary element of international collaboration there generally has to be international co-ordination as well, usually under an appropriate political umbrella. Although such issues have not yet surfaced for PPR it might still be possible make progress in eradicating the virus from countries on the borders of its geographical distribution. If the appropriate preliminary surveys were undertaken to delineate the infected areas, there is no reason why vaccination campaigns should not be permanently successful in countries such as Turkey, Syria, Jordan and Egypt. In such situations, if pulsed vaccination campaigns were to be contemplated, it would be worth considering administering the vaccine as part of a cocktail, either using antigens derived from several different conventional vaccines, or a bioengineered product whereby the major small ruminant pathogens of a given country were all attacked simultaneously.

11.13 Conclusions

In general the use of vaccines presents as many problems relating to the design and innovation of new strategies as it does the need for novel vaccines.

References

Anderson,J., McKay,J.A. & Butcher,R.N. 1991 The use of monoclonal antibodies in competitive Elisa for the detection of antibodies to rinderpest and peste des petits ruminants viruses. In "The seromonitoring of rinderpest throughout Africa. Phase 1".IAEA-Tecdoc-623, International Atomic Energy Agency, Vienna pp 43-53

Anderson,J., Anderson,E.C., Chiduo,F., Joshua,G.E., Loretu,K., Mpelumbe,I.E. & Kavishe,T.E. 1991 Field evaluation of the indirect ELISA for seromonitoring during the rinderpest eradication campaign in Tanzania. .In "The sero-monitoring of rinderpest throughout Africa; Phase 1". IAEA-Techdoc-623, International Atomic Energy Agency, Vienna. pp 87-109.

Atang,P.G. & Plowright,W. 1969 Extension of the JP15 rinderpest control campaign to eastern Africa the epizootiological background. Bull.epiz.Dis.Afr. 17 161-170.

Barrett,T., Forsyth,M., Inui,K., Wamwayi,H.M., Kock,R., Wambua,J., Mwanzia,J. & Rossiter,P.B. 1998 Rediscovery of the second African lineage of rinderpest virus: its epidemiological significance. Vet.Rec. 142 669-671.

Branagan,D & Hammond,J. 1965 Rinderpest in Tanganyika: A review. Bull.epiz.Dis.Afr. 13 225-246.

Brown,C.C. 1997 A review of three pathology-based techniques for retrospective diagnosis of rinderpest, with comparison to virus isolation. Res.Vet.Sci. 63 103-106.

Brown,R.D. 1958 Rinderpest immunity in calves. I. The acquisition and persistence of maternally derived antibody. J.Hyg.,Camb. 56 427-434.

Diallo,A., Barrett,T., Subbarao,S.M & Taylor,W.P. 1989 Differentiation of rinderpest and *peste des petits ruminants* viruses using cDNA clones. Journal of Virological methods 23 127-137.

El Hag Ali,B. 1973 A natural outbreak of rinderpest involving sheep, goats and cattle in Sudan. Bull.epiz.Dis.Afr. 21 421-428.

Felsenstein,J. 1990 Phylip Manual Version 3.3. University Herbarium, University of California, Berkeley, California.

Foreman,A.J., Rowe,L.W. & Taylor,W.P. 1983 Detection of rinderpest antigen by agar gel immunodiffusion and counter-immunoelectrophoresis. Trop.Anim.Hlth.Prod. 15 83-85.

Forsyth,M. & Barrett,T. 1995 Evaluation of polymerase chain reaction for the detection and characterisation of rinderpest and peste des petits ruminants viruses for epidemiological studies. Virus Research 39 151-163.

Govindarajan,R., Koteeswaran,A., Venugopalan,A.T., Shyam,G., Shaquna,S., Shaila,M.S. & Ramachandran,S. 1997 Isolation of peste des petits ruminants virus from an outbreak in Indian Buffalo (Bubalus bubalis) Vet.Rec. 141 573-574.

Libeau,G., Colas,F & Guerre,L. 1994 Rapid differential diagnosis of rinderpest and peste des petits ruminants using an immunocapture ELISA. Vet.Rec. 134 300-304.

Liess,B. & Plowright,W. 1964 Studies on the pathogenesis of rinderpest in experimental cattle. I. Correlation of clinical signs, viraemia and virus excretion by various routes. J.Hyg.,Camb. 62 81-100.

Littlewood,W. 1905 Cattle plague in Egypt in 1903-04-05. J.Comp.Path. 18 312-321.

Macadam,I. 1968 Transmission of rinderpest from goats to cattle in Tanzania. Bull.epiz.Dis.Afr. 16 53-60.

Mariner,J.C., House,J.A., Sollod,A.E., Stem,C., van den Ende,M.C. & Mebus,C.A. 1990 Comparison of the effect of various chemical stabilisers and lyophilisation cycles on the thermostability of a Vero cell-adapted rinderpest vaccine. Vet.Microbiol. 21 195 - 209.

Maurer,F.D., Jones,T.C., Easterday,B. & DeTray,D. 1955 Proceedings of the 92nd Annual Meeting of the American Veterinary Medical Association 201-211.

Nawathe,D.R. & Lamorde,A.G. 1984 Socio-economic impact of rinderpest in Nigeria. Rev.sci.tech.Off.int.Epiz. 3 575-581.

Office International des Epizooties (OIE) 1998 Guide to epidemiological surveillance for rinderpest. Rev.sci.tech.Off.int.Epiz., 17 796-824.

Office International des Epizooties (OIE) 1996 Manual of Standards for Diagnostic tests and Vaccines, 3rd Edition, Office International des Epizooties, Paris.

Plowright,W. 1964 Studies on the pathogenesis of rinderpest in experimental cattle. II. Proliferation of the virus in different tissues following intranasal infection. J.Hyg.,Camb. 62 257-281.

Plowright,W. 1998 The global professional commitment to the success of the Global rinderpest Eradication Programme. FAO Technical Consultation on the Global Rinderpest Eradication Programme, FAO, Rome.

Plowright,W. & Taylor,W.P. 1967 Long-term studies of the immunity in East African cattle following inoculation with rinderpest culture vaccine. Res.vet.Sci. 8 118-128.

Robson,J., Arnold,R.M., Plowright,W. & Scott,G.R. 1959 The isolation from an eland of a strain of rinderpest virus attenuated for cattle. Bull.epiz.Dis.Afr. 7 97-102.

Rossiter,P.B., Jessett,D.M., Wafula,J.S., Karsted,L., Chema,S., Taylor,W.P., Rowe,L., Nyange, J.C., Otaru,M., Mumbala,M. & Scott,G.R. 1983 Re-emergence of rinderpest as a threat in East Africa since 1979. Vet.Rec. 113 459-461.

Salem-Bey,I.F. 1947 Cattle plague in Egypt. Ministry of Agriculture, Egypt. Technical and Scientific Service Bulletin No. 88. pp 1-47.

Taylor,W.P. & Nanda,Y.P. 1995 Rinderpest: Towards eradication. Comprehensive reports on technical items presented to the International Committee or to Regional Commissions. OIE, Paris. pp 97-100.

Taylor,W.P. & Plowright,W. 1965 Studies on the pathogenesis of rinderpest in experimental cattle. III. Proliferation of an attenuated strain in various tissues following subcutaneous inoculation. J.Hyg.,Camb. 63 263-275.

Taylor,W.P. & Watson,R.M. 1967 Studies on the epizootiology of rinderpest in blue wildebeest and other game species of Northern Tanzania and Southern Kenya, 1965 -7. J.Hyg.,Camb. 65 537-545.

Taylor,W.P., Plowright,W., Pillinger,R. Rampton,C.S. & Staple,R. 1965 Studies on the pathogenesis of rinderpest in experimental cattle. IV. Proliferation of the virus following contact infection. J.Hyg.,Camb. 63 497-506.

Tyler,L. 1991 PARC sero-monitoring: Survey design, implementation and the analysis, presentation and use of results. In "The sero-monitoring of rinderpest throughout Africa; Phase 1". IAEA-Techdoc-623, International |Atomic Energy Agency, Vienna. pp 87-109.

Wohlsein,P., Trautwein,G., Harder,T.C., Leiss,B. & Barrett,T. 1993 Viral antigen distribution in organs of cattle experimentally infected with rinderpest virus. Vet.Pathol. 30 544-554.

Wohlsein,P., Wamwayi,H.M., Trautwein,G., Pohlenz,J., Leiss,B. & Barrett,T. 1995 Pathomorphological and immunohistological findings in cattle experimentally infected with rinderpest virus isolates of different pathogenicity. Vet.Microbiol 44 141 - 147.

Appendix 2

A Glossary of Common Epidemiological and Economic Terms

Accuracy - the degree to which a measurement, or an estimate based on measurements, represents the true value of the attribute that is being measured. See also "Precsion" and "Validity" which are the two components of "Accuracy".

Agent - a factor such as a microorganism or chemical substance whose presence or excessive presence is necessary for the occurrence of a disease.

Analysis of variance - also called ANOVA; a statistical technique that isolates and assesses the contribution of categorical variables, each with more than 2 classes, to variation in the mean of a continuous variable. See also t-test.

Analytical Sensitivity - The ability of a laboratory assay to detect small amounts of the target substance. This is a laboratory term which is equivalent to the epidemiological term, "sensitivity" which is sometimes called "population sensitivity". An equivalent term for "specificity" is sometimes used.

Analytical study - a hypothesis testing method of investigating the association between a given disease, health state, or other outcome variable, and possible causative factors.

Association - the degree of statistical dependence between two or more events or variables. Events are said to be associated when they occur more frequently together than one would expect by chance. Association does not necessarily imply a causal relationship. Statistical significance testing enables us to determine how unlikely it would be to observe the sample relationship by chance if in fact no relationship exists in the population that was sampled.

Attributable Risk - the excess risk (above background) that is explained by the characteristic or risk factor under study. It requires calculation of incidence rates.

$$\textit{Attributable risk} = \textit{Incidence rate}_{exp} - \textit{Incidence rate}_{non\text{-}exp}$$

Attack Rate - the proportion of a specific population affected during an outbreak. The population is usually limited to susceptible animals or those identifiably at risk. It is a special form of cumulative incidence that is used in an outbreak investigation.

Benefit-Cost Ratio - the ratio of the net present values (usually monetary values) of measurable benefits to costs. Used to determine the economic feasibility or probability of success of a time-bounded program.

Bias - any effect at any stage of an investigation tending to produce results that depart systematically from the true values i.e. a systematic error.

Bias (Response bias) - a systematic error due to differences in characteristics between those who volunteer to participate in a study and those who do not.

Bias (Selection bias) - error due to systematic differences in characteristics between those animals or herds which are selected for study and those which are not.

Bimodal Distribution - a distribution with two regions of high frequency separated by a region of low frequency of observation.

Binomial Distribution - a probability distribution associated with two mutually exclusive outcomes such as yes or no.

Carrier - an animal which is capable of transmitting infection but shows no clinical signs. A carrier can be incubatory, convalescent, or chronic.

Case-Control Study - a study that starts with the identification of animals (or herds) with the disease of interest and a suitable control (comparison, reference) group of animals (or herds) without the disease. This type of study involves collection and analysis of data on disease determinants in the two groups. Usually, it is a retrospective study because disease events have occurred before the exposure history is determined.

Case-Fatality Rate - the proportion of animals contracting a disease that die of that disease during a specified follow-up period.

$$\textit{Case-fatality rate} = \frac{\textit{No. of deaths from specific cause}}{\textit{No. cases of specific cause}}$$

Categorical Data - qualitative data which can be allocated to specific groups. May be nominal (ie. named) or ordinal (ie. ordered) or dichotomous (ie. presence/absence).

Cause, Necessary - a variable which must always precede an effect. This effect need not be a sole result of the one variable.

Chain of Infection - the series of mechanisms by which an infectious organism passes from an infected to a susceptible host as shown in the diagram below (see also Method of Transmission).

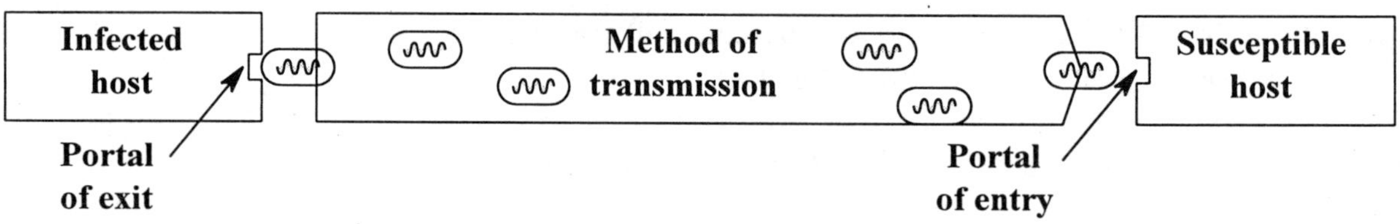

Chi-Square Test - a method of testing to determine whether two or more series of proportions or frequencies are significantly different from one another or whether a single series of proportions differs significantly from an expected distribution. Pearson's Chi-square is used for unmatched data and McNemar's Chi-square for matched data. See definition of association for further explanation.

Clustering - a closely grouped series of events or cases of a disease in relation to time or place or both. The term is normally used to describe aggregation of relatively uncommon events or diseases.

Cohort Study - An epidemiologic study in which subsets of a defined population are sampled on the basis of exposure to a factor or factors hypothesized to influence the probability of occurrence of a given disease or other outcome. It is commonly undertaken prospectively.

Conceptual Model - a representation of a system or process, usually in diagramatic form which shows important relationships among the different elements (see also Mathematical Model).

Confidence Limits - an interval whose end points can be calculated from observational data and has a specified probability of containing the parameter of interest.

Confounding - a situation in which the effects of two factors are not separated. The distortion of the apparent effect of an exposure or risk factor brought about by association with other factors that can influence the outcome.

Confounding Factor - a confounding factor or variable is one which is distributed non-randomly with respect to the independent (exposure) variable and is associated with the dependent (outcome) variable being studied. The association with the dependent variable is usually established from results of previous studies.

Contagious - Transmitted by direct contact. (See also "Transmission of Infection")

Contingency Table - a tabular cross-classification of data such that subcategories of one characteristic are indicated horizontally (in rows) and subcategories of another characteristic are indicated vertically (in columns), and the number of units in each cell is indicated. The simplest contingency table is the fourfold or 2 x 2 table, but a contingency table may include several dimensions of classification.

Continuous Data - quantitative data with a potentially infinite number of possible values along a continuum.

Correlation Coefficient - a measure of association that indicates the degree to which two or more sets of observations fit a linear relationship. This coefficient, represented by the letter "r", can vary between +1 and -1. If "r" is +1, there is a perfect linear relationship in which one variable varies directly with the other. If "r" = -1, there is again a perfect linear association but one variable varies inversely with the other.

Cost Benefit Analysis - methods of identifying the losses and gains in monetary terms of the effects of a disease that are incurred by society as a whole.

Cross-Sectional Study - (syn: prevalence study) - a study carried out on a representative sample of a population that examines the relationship between a disease or other health-related characteristic and other variables of interest as they exist in a defined population at one particular time.

Crude Rate - a rate which applies to a total population irrespective of the attributes of that population (cf. specific rate).

Data - facts of any kind. Data are plural, datum is singular.

Database - a systemised collection of information, commonly on electronic media about a specific subject such as animal disease.

Decision Analysis - application of probability theory with the aim of calculating the optimal strategy from a series of alternative decisions which are often expressed graphically in the form of a decision tree. Decision analysis is a tool to help stock owners decide which of several options eg vaccination or culling is the optimal alternative for treatment or control of a disease.

Denominator - the population at risk in the calculation of a rate or ratio. See also Numerator

Dependent Variable - (syn:outcome/response variable) a variable or factor, the value of which depends on or is hypothesized to depend on the effect of other [causal] variable(s) in the study.

Determinant - any factor whether event, characteristic or other definable entity, that brings about change in a health condition or other defined characteristic.

Deterministic Model - a mathematical model which assumes all parameters and variables are constant and not random variables.

Diagnostic test - a test or procedure applied to a diseased individual. (See also "Screening" and "Screening Test")

Disease Determinant - any variable (factor) associated with a disease which if removed or altered results in a change in the incidence of disease in a population.

Disease Reservoir - any animal or object in which an infectious agent multiplies or develops and upon which it depends as a species for survival in nature.

Discriminant Analysis - a statistical technique similar to regression analysis but where the response, or dependent variable is dichotomous. Alternatively - a statistical method used to allocate an individual to one or more distinct groups.

Dose-Response Relationship - a relationship in which change in amount, intensity or duration of exposure to a factor is associated with a change (either an increase or a decrease) in risk of a specified outcome.

Endemic Disease - the constant presence of a disease or infectious agent within a given geographic area or population group. It also implies a prevalence which is usual in the area or in the population.

Epidemic - the occurrence in a population or region of cases of disease clearly in excess of normal expectancy. Epidemics in a large population often occur as smaller epidemics in separate subdivisions of the overall population. In general, these smaller epidemics are not in phase but interact with each other to some extent.

Epidemic curve - a histogram in which the X-axis represents the time of occurrence of disease cases and the Y-axis represents the frequency of disease cases. It is a useful tool to determine the epidemiology of disease occurrence in an outbreak investigation.

Epidemic, Propagating - an outbreak or series of outbreaks resulting from animal to animal spread.

Epidemiology - the study of the distribution and determinants of health related states and events in populations. It is a term now in common usage for studies in animal populations although epizootiology is still occasionally used.

Epidemiology, Descriptive - study of the occurrence of disease or other health related characteristics in populations. Implies general observation rather than analysis.

Error, Sampling - after testing a sample from a large population, the mean or any other statistic calculated from the sample will have a different value from the true value if the whole population was measured. The difference between the value for the whole population and its estimate calculated from the sample is called the sampling error.

Error, Systematic - that due to factors other than chance, such as faulty measuring instruments.

Experimental Epidemiology - the planning of specific population experiments to test epidemiological hypotheses (eg field trials, clinical trials).

Experimental Study - a study in which the conditions are under the direct control of the investigator.

False Negative - when the result of an individual test is negative but the disease or condition is present.

False Positive - when the result of an individual test is positive but the disease or condition is not present.

Frequency - a count, or number of occurrences, of an event in a specified population and time period.

Frequency Distribution - any arrangement of numerical data obtained by measuring a parameter in a population.

Histogram - frequency distribution plotted in the form of rectangles whose bases are equal to the class width and whose areas are proportional to the absolute or relative frequencies.

Herd immunity - the resistance of a group of animals to invasion and spread of an infectious agent based on the resistance to infection of a high proportion (but not all) members of the group. Also called "population immunity"

Hypotheses - a proposition that can be tested by facts that are known or can be obtained. The assertion that an association between two, or more variables or a difference between 2 or more groups, exists in the larger population of interest.

Immunity - the resistance of an individual to infection or disease due to a particular agent. Immunity may be innate (natural), passive (eg maternal or through administration of immune serum), or active from previous exposure or vaccination.

Incidence - the number of new cases of disease or other condition which occur in a specified population during a given period. Mathematically, 2 types of incidence rate can be distinguished. These are incidence density rate and cumulative incidence.

Incubation Period - the interval of time from exposure to infection through to when clinical signs are first manifested in an individual.

Independent Variable - the characteristic being observed or measured that is hypothesized to influence an event. An independent variable is not influenced by the event or manifestation but may cause it or contribute to its variation.

Index Case - the first diagnosed case of an outbreak in a herd or other defined group.

Infectivity - the ability of an agent to enter, survive and multiply in a susceptible host. Epidemiologically, it is measured as the proportion of the individuals exposed to an agent who become infected. See also "pathogenicity" and "virulence".

Inference - the process of passing from observations to generalisations.

Intervention Study - an epidemiologic investigation designed to test a hypothesized cause-effect relationship by modifying a supposed causal factor in a population and measuring the change in the parameter.

Latent Infection - persistence of an infectious agent within the host without symptoms of disease.

Linear Regression - statistical method used to study the relationship between independent and dependent variables when the dependent variable consists of continuous data.

Log-Linear Model - a statistical model that uses an analysis of variance type of approach for the modelling of frequency counts in contingency tables.

Longitudinal Study - a study conducted over a defined period of time which may be either retrospective or prospective. See also Case Control and Cohort Study.

Marginal cost (of animal health) - the cost of an additional amount of animal health care.

Marginal Return (of animal health) - the income obtained from using an additional amount of animal health care.

Matching - the process of making a study group and a comparison group comparable with respect to factors which are likely to influence the results but in which the experimenter has no immediate interest.

Mathematical Model - a representation of a system or process in mathematical form in which equations are used to simulate the behavior of the system or process under study (see also Conceptual Model).

Mean-Arithmetic - a measure of central tendency computed by adding all the individual values together and dividing by the number in the group.

Mean-Geometric - a measure of central tendency calculable only for positive values and computed by taking the logarithms of the values, calculating their arithmetic mean and then converting back to the original units by taking the antilogarithms.

Median - the median is the middle value of a set of observations arranged in order of magnitude.

Mode - the mode is the most frequently occurring value in a set of observations. A given set of observations can have more than one mode. (see also Bimodal Distribution).

Method of Transmission - see Transmission of Infection

Model - a representation or simulation of an actual situation.

Monitoring - observation of an infected population aimed at measuring changes in the prevalence or incidence of disease. Often used to chart progress of a disease control program in assessing its effectiveness. (See also "Surveillance")

Multiple Regression - an analytical method which determines the relationship between a dependent variable and two or more independent variables.

Multistage Sampling - a term applied to the selection of a sample in two or more stages. eg, selecting a sample of herds and then a sample of livestock within those herds.

Multivariate Analysis - a set of techniques used when the variation in several variables has to be studied simultaneously. In statistics, any analytic method that allows the simultaneous study of two or more dependent variables.

Natural History of Disease - the progress of a disease in an individual animal over time without intervention as it occurs in the natural rather than a controlled situation such as in a laboratory or pen experiment. For convenience, the continuum of the natural history of a disease is simplified into a number of discrete states through which an individual progresses with time. This is shown below:

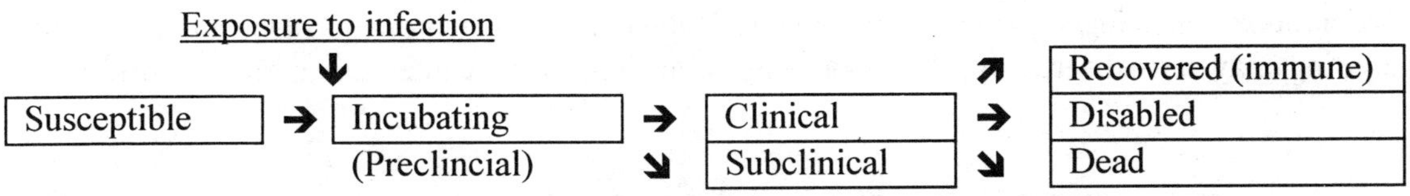

A **convalescent** state is sometimes included to denote an individual who no longer has clinical signs but has not yet returned to full function and production. Depending on the particular disease, recovered animals may remain immune for life or revert to susceptibility over time.

Necessary Cause - the characteristic referred to as the "cause" which is always found in the presence of the effect.

Nominal Data - a type of data in which there are limited categories but no order, such as breed and eye color.

Normal - within the usual range of variation in a given population or population group; or frequently occurring in a given population or group.

Normal Distribution - a continuous symmetrical frequency distribution where both tails extend to infinity, the arithmetic mean, mode and median are identical. Graphically it is a bell shaped curve and its steepness or shape is completely determined by the mean and variance.

Null Hypothesis - the hypothesis that two variables have no association at all, or two or more population distributions do not differ from each other.

Numerator - the upper portion of a fraction used to calculate a rate or ratio.

Observational Study - an epidemiological study where nature is allowed to take its course while changes or differences in one characteristic are studied in relation to changes or differences in other(s) without intervention of the investigator (e.g. descriptive, cross-sectional case-control, cohort).

Occurrence - a statement indicating the presence of disease without signifying the frequency. This definition describes the use of the word in international animal disease reports.

Odds Ratio - the ratio of two odds. In a case-control study, the ratio of the odds of exposure among the cases to the odds of exposure among the non-cases. In a cohort or cross sectional study, the ratio of the odds of disease in the exposed to the odds of disease in the unexposed. Mathematically, the odds ratio is calculated identically for all types of study design.

	Diseased	Not diseased
Exposed	**a**	**b**
Unexposed	**c**	**d**

The Odds Ratio is ad/bc

Ordinal data - a type of data in which there are limited categories with an inherent ranking from lowest to highest (such as severity of disease).

Outbreak - the occurrence of disease in an identifiable group of animals at a level greater than that normally expected. For practical purposes, the term is synonymous with a short term epidemic. (See also "Epidemic")

Outliers - observations differing so widely from the rest of the data as to lead one to suspect that a gross error in recording may have been committed, or suggesting that these values came from a different population.

Pandemic - an epidemic occurring over a very wide area, involving many countries and usually affecting a large proportion of the population.

Parameter - a summary descriptive characteristic of a population (cf statistic - which is a sample-based measure).

Pathogenicity - the ability of an organism to produce disease regardless of its level of severity. Epidemiologically, it is measured as the proportion of infected individuals who develop clinical disease. See also "infectivity" and "virulence".

Population - A defined group whose individual members have the potential to interact with one another and can be distinguished from other groups.

Power - probability of finding a difference between two or more groups given that a difference exists. Power = 1-Beta = 1-Probability of a type II error.

Precision - the quality of being sharply defined or stated. Refers to the ability of a test or measuring device to give consistent results when applied repeatedly. Sometimes also called "repeatability". See also "validity". A good test is both precise and valid which are the two components of accuracy.

Predictive Value - in screening or diagnostic tests, the predictive value of a positive test is the proportion of test positive animals that have the disease. The predictive value of a negative test is the probability that an animal with a negative test does not have the disease. The predictive value of a test is determined by the sensitivity and specificity of the test, and by the prevalence of the condition at the time the test is used.

Prevalence - the proportion of cases of a disease or other condition present in a population without any distinction between old and new cases. When used without qualification the term usually refers to the number of cases as a proportion of the population at risk at a specified point in time (point prevalence).

$$\textit{Prevalence} = \frac{\textit{No. cases at specific point in time}}{\textit{Population at risk at same point in time}}$$

Prevalence study - see cross-sectional study

Primary Case - the individual that introduces disease into a herd, flock, or other group under study. Not necessarily the first diagnosed case in that herd. See index case.

Proportion - a fraction where the numerator is a subset of the denominator.

Prospective Study - see Cohort Study.

Qualitative data - that which possess specific qualities such as breed, gender, or color. See nominal data.

Random - governed by chance.

Randomisation - allocation of individuals to groups by chance. Within the limits of chance variation, randomization should make control and experimental groups similar at the start of an investigation and ensure that personal judgement and prejudices of the investigator do not influence allocation. Note that random allocation follows a predetermined plan often devised with the aid of a table of random numbers or by an electronic random number generator.

Random Sample - a sample of a population assembled so that each member of the population has an equal and non-zero opportunity to be selected.

Random Statistic - a sampling procedure for selecting individuals from a population so that each has an equal chance of being selected in the sample.

Rate - an expression of the change in one quantity per unit time.
It is a ratio whose essential characteristic is that time is an element of the denominator and in which there is a distinct relationship between numerator and denominator. See also ratio and proportion.

Ratio - the expression of the relationship between a numerator and denominator where the two are separate and distinct quantities, i.e the numerator is not included in the denominator.

Regression Analysis - a statistical technique used to examine the relationship between two continuous variables. See also linear regression.

Relative Risk - the ratio of the disease incidence in individuals exposed to a hypothesized factor to the incidence in individuals not exposed; a measure of association commonly used in cohort studies. See also odds ratio.

	Diseased	Not diseased
Exposed	**a**	**b**
Unexposed	**c**	**d**

The Relative Risk is $[a/(a+b)] \div [c/(c+d)]$

Repeatability - the ability of a test to give consistent results in repeated tests. See precision.

Replication - the execution of an experiment or survey more than once to confirm the findings and obtain an improved estimate of sampling error.

Response Rate - the number of completed or returned survey instruments (questionnaires. interview etc.) divided by the total number of individuals selected for study.

Retrospective Study - a study that collects and utilizes historical data. A case-control study is retrospective because it looks back from the point of known effects to determine causative factors.

Risk Factor - an attribute or exposure that increases the probability of occurrence of disease or other specified outcome.

Sampling - the process of selecting a number of representative subjects from all the subjects in a particular group. Conclusions based on sample results may be attributed only to the population sampled. See also random sample and selection bias.

Screening - implies subjecting an apparently healthy population or sample of a population to a test or procedure, with the objective of detecting disease. Tests used for this purpose are usually cheap, easily performed, sensitive but often not very specific. (See also "Screening" and "Diagnostic Test")

Screening test - a test or procedure applied to an apparently healthy individual. (See also "Screening" and "Diagnostic Test")

Secular trend - a long term trend in the occurrence of disease or other condition.

Sensitivity (synonym: True Positive Rate): The proportion of animals with the disease (or infection) of interest who test positive. It is a measure of the probability that a diseased individual will be correctly identified by the test. Sometimes called "population sensitivity" to distinguish from "analytical sensitivity".

Sentinel Herds - herds that are reasonably representative of the population as a whole and which are tested at regular intervals for infectious disease to determine whether and to what extent the diseases are occurring in the population.

Seroepidemiology - epidemiological studies based on an examination of sera taken from the population or a sample of the population.

Significance, Level of - also known as alpha (a) or type I error rate. The probability of saying a difference exists when none does.

Spatial distribution - the relationship of disease events to location of individual animals or clusters of animals.

Specificity (synonym: True Negative Rate) - the proportion of animals without the disease (or infection) of interest who test negative. It is a measure of the probability that an individual without the disease of interest will be correctly identified by the test. Sometimes called "population specificity" to distinguish from "analytical specificity".

Specific Rate - expresses the frequency of a characteristic per unit size of a specific population.

Sporadic - a disease occurring irregularly and generally infrequently and without any apparent underlying pattern.

Standard Deviation - a measure of dispersion or variation. Equal to the positive square root of the variance. The mean indicates where the values for a group are centered. The standard deviation is a measure of how widely values are dispersed around the mean in the population.

Standard Error - measure of the variability of a sample statistic that specifically relates an observed mean to the true mean of the population.

summary value calculated from a sample of observations usually to estimate a population parameter.

Statistical Significance - statistical methods allow an estimate to be made of the probability of the observed degree of association between independent and dependent variables being exceeded under a null hypothesis. From this estimate the statistical "significance" of a result can be stated. Usually the level of statistical significance is stated by the "P" value or probability value. See also Significance, Level of.

Statistics - the science and art of dealing with variation in data through collection, classification, and appropriate analysis.

Stochastic Model - a mathematical model which takes into consideration the presence of variability in one or more of its parameters.

Stratified Sample - involves dividing the population into distinct subgroups according to some important characteristic, eg herd size, and selecting a random sample out of each subgroup.

Spread of infection - the movement of infection from an infected population or subdivision of a population to a susceptible population or subdivision. See also "Transmission of Infection".

Surveillance - observation of a susceptible (uninfected) population aimed at the early detection of cases of a particular disease so that control action can be quickly instituted. (See also "Monitoring")

Surveillance is often subdivided into two categories, **passive** and **active**.

Passive surveillance is the **secondary use** of routinely collected data which was generated for some other purpose such a diagnostic service.
Active surveillance is the routine collection of data whose **primary purpose** is for surveillance.

Survey - an investigation in which information is systematically collected.

Systematic Sample - the procedure of selecting according to some simple systematic rule, such as every 5th cow in the herd as they enter the milking parlor. A systematic sample may lead to errors that invalidate generalizations.

Temporal Distribution - the relationship of disease events to time.

Theoretical Epidemiology - the development of mathematical/statistical models to explain different aspects of the occurrence of a variety of diseases.

Transmission of infection - the carriage of an infectious agent from an infective to a susceptible individual within an infected population or subdivision of a population. See also "spread". The different modes (methods) of transmission are summarised in the following table:

Direct transmission		**Indirect transmission**	
Contact		Airborne	- droplet nuclei (<5 microns)
			- dust (>5 microns)
Droplet		Vehicle	(fomites)
Vertical	- in-utero	Vector	- mechanical
	- milk		- biological

Trend - a long-time movement in an ordered series (e.g. a time series). An essential feature is that the movement, whilst possibly irregular in the short term, shows movement consistently in the same direction over a long term.

T test - a test where data is continuous, and there are two comparison groups. It can be used to (1) estimate the mean of a normally distributed population, or to (2) test the difference between two sample means. See also analysis of variance.

Type I Error - an error which occurs when using data from a sample that demonstrates a statistically significant association when no such association is present in the population. Equals the level of significance or alpha.

Type II Error - an error that occurs from failure to demonstrate a statistically significant association when one exists in a population. Equals Beta. The power of a study equals 1-Beta.

Validity - the extent to which a study or test measures what it sets out to measure. See also "precision". A good test is both precise and valid which are the two components of accuracy.

Variable - see Dependent variable, Independent variable.

Variance - the variance of a set of observations is the sum of squares of the deviation of each observation from the arithmetic mean of the observations, divided by one less than the number of observations.

Vector - a living organism (frequently an arthropod) that transports an infectious agent from an infected animal or its wastes to a susceptible individual, its food or immediate surroundings. Vectors may be **mechanical** through external contamination or passage of the agent through the gastrointestinal tract or **biological** where propagation (multiplication), cyclic development or a combination (cyclopropagation) is required before the vector can transmit the infective form of the agent.

Virulence - the degree of severity of disease produced by an agent in a given host. Epidemiologically, it is measured as the proportion of individuals with disease who become seriously ill or die. The case-fatality rate is a measure of virulence. See also "infectivity" and "virulence".

FAO ANIMAL PRODUCTION AND HEALTH PAPERS

1 Animal breeding: selected articles from the *World Animal Review*, 1977 (C E F S)
2 Eradication of hog cholera and African swine fever, 1976 (E F S)
3 Insecticides and application equipment for tsetse control, 1977 (E F)
4 New feed resources, 1977 (E/F/S)
5 Bibliography of the criollo cattle of the Americas, 1977 (E/S)
6 Mediterranean cattle and sheep in crossbreeding, 1977 (E F)
7 The environmental impact of tsetse control operations, 1977 (E F)
7 Rev. 1 The environmental impact of tsetse control operations, 1980 (E F)
8 Declining breeds of Mediterranean sheep, 1978 (E F)
9 Slaughterhouse and slaughterslab design and construction, 1978 (E F S)
10 Treating straw for animal feeding, 1978 (C E F S)
11 Packaging, storage and distribution of processed milk, 1978 (E)
12 Ruminant nutrition: selected articles from the *World Animal Review*, 1978 (C E F S)
13 Buffalo reproduction and artificial insemination, 1979 (E*)
14 The African trypanosomiases, 1979 (E F)
15 Establishment of dairy training centres, 1979 (E)
16 Open yard housing for young cattle, 1981 (Ar E F S)
17 Prolific tropical sheep, 1980 (E F S)
18 Feed from animal wastes: state of knowledge, 1980 (C E)
19 East Coast fever and related tick-borne diseases, 1980 (E)
20/1 Trypanotolerant livestock in West and Central Africa – Vol. 1. General study, 1980 (E F)
20/2 Trypanotolerant livestock in West and Central Africa – Vol. 2. Country studies, 1980 (E F)
20/3 Le bétail trypanotolérant en Afrique occidentale et centrale – Vol. 3. Bilan d'une décennie, 1988 (F)
21 Guideline for dairy accounting, 1980 (E)
22 Recursos genéticos animales en América Latina, 1981 (S)
23 Disease control in semen and embryos, 1981 (C E F S)
24 Animal genetic resources – conservation and management, 1981 (C E)
25 Reproductive efficiency in cattle, 1982 (C E F S)
26 Camels and camel milk, 1982 (E)
27 Deer farming, 1982 (E)
28 Feed from animal wastes: feeding manual, 1982 (C E)
29 Echinococcosis/hydatidosis surveillance, prevention and control: FAO/UNEP/WHO guidelines, 1982 (E)
30 Sheep and goat breeds of India, 1982 (E)
31 Hormones in animal production, 1982 (E)
32 Crop residues and agro-industrial by-products in animal feeding, 1982 (E/F)
33 Haemorrhagic septicaemia, 1982 (E F)
34 Breeding plans for ruminant livestock in the tropics, 1982 (E F S)
35 Off-tastes in raw and reconstituted milk, 1983 (Ar E F S)
36 Ticks and tick-borne diseases: selected articles from the *World Animal Review*, 1983 (E F S)
37 African animal trypanosomiasis: selected articles from the *World Animal Review*, 1983 (E F)
38 Diagnosis and vaccination for the control of brucellosis in the Near East, 1982 (Ar E)
39 Solar energy in small-scale milk collection and processing, 1983 (E F)
40 Intensive sheep production in the Near East, 1983 (Ar E)
41 Integrating crops and livestock in West Africa, 1983 (E F)
42 Animal energy in agriculture in Africa and Asia, 1984 (E/F S)
43 Olive by-products for animal feed, 1985 (Ar E F S)
44/1 Animal genetic resources conservation by management, data banks and training, 1984 (E)
44/2 Animal genetic resources: cryogenic storage of germplasm and molecular engineering, 1984 (E)
45 Maintenance systems for the dairy plant, 1984 (E)
46 Livestock breeds of China, 1984 (E F S)
47 Réfrigération du lait à la ferme et organisation des transports, 1985 (F)
48 La fromagerie et les variétés de fromages du bassin méditerranéen, 1985 (F)
49 Manual for the slaughter of small ruminants in developing countries, 1985 (E)
50 Better utilization of crop residues and by-products in animal feeding: research guidelines – 1. State of knowledge, 1985 (E)
50/2 Better utilization of crop residues and by-products in animal feeding: research guidelines – 2. A practical manual for research workers, 1986 (E)
51 Dried salted meats: charque and carne-de-sol, 1985 (E)
52 Small-scale sausage production, 1985 (E)
53 Slaughterhouse cleaning and sanitation, 1985 (E)
54 Small ruminants in the Near East – Vol. I. Selected papers presented for the Expert Consultation on Small Ruminant Research and Development in the Near East (Tunis, 1985), 1987 (E)
55 Small ruminants in the Near East – Vol. II. Selected articles from *World Animal Review* 1972-1986, 1987 (Ar E)
56 Sheep and goats in Pakistan, 1985 (E)
57 The Awassi sheep with special reference to the improved dairy type, 1985 (E)
58 Small ruminant production in the developing countries, 1986 (E)
59/1 Animal genetic resources data banks – 1. Computer systems study for regional data banks, 1986 (E)
59/2 Animal genetic resources data banks – 2. Descriptor lists for cattle, buffalo, pigs, sheep and goats, 1986 (E F S)
59/3 Animal genetic resources data banks – 3. Descriptor lists for poultry, 1986 (E F S)
60 Sheep and goats in Turkey, 1986 (E)
61 The Przewalski horse and restoration to its natural habitat in Mongolia, 1986 (E)
62 Milk and dairy products: production and processing costs, 1988 (E F S)
63 Proceedings of the FAO expert consultation on the substitution of imported concentrate feeds in animal production systems in developing countries, 1987 (C E)
64 Poultry management and diseases in the Near East, 1987 (Ar)
65 Animal genetic resources of the USSR, 1989 (E)
66 Animal genetic resources – strategies for improved use and conservation, 1987 (E)
67/1 Trypanotolerant cattle and livestock development in West and Central Africa – Vol. I, 1987 (E)
67/2 Trypanotolerant cattle and livestock development in West and Central Africa – Vol. II, 1987 (E)

68 Crossbreeding *Bos indicus* and *Bos taurus* for milk production in the tropics, 1987 (E)
69 Village milk processing, 1988 (E F S)
70 Sheep and goat meat production in the humid tropics of West Africa, 1989 (E/F)
71 The development of village-based sheep production in West Africa, 1988 (Ar E F S)
(Published as Training manual for extension workers, M/S5840E)
72 Sugarcane as feed, 1988 (E/S)
73 Standard design for small-scale modular slaughterhouses, 1988 (E)
74 Small ruminants in the Near East – Vol. III. North Africa, 1989 (E)
75 The eradication of ticks, 1989 (E/S)
76 *Ex situ* cryoconservation of genomes and genes of endangered cattle breeds by means of modern biotechnological methods, 1989 (E)
77 Training manual for embryo transfer in cattle, 1991 (E)
78 Milking, milk production hygiene and udder health, 1989 (E)
79 Manual of simple methods of meat preservation, 1990 (E)
80 Animal genetic resources – a global programme for sustainable development, 1990 (E)
81 Veterinary diagnostic bacteriology – a manual of laboratory procedures of selected diseases of livestock, 1990 (E F)
82 Reproduction in camels – a review, 1990 (E)
83 Training manual on artificial insemination in sheep and goats, 1991 (E F)
84 Training manual for embryo transfer in water buffaloes, 1991 (E)
85 The technology of traditional milk products in developing countries, 1990 (E)
86 Feeding dairy cows in the tropics, 1991 (E)
87 Manual for the production of anthrax and blackleg vaccines, 1991 (E F)
88 Small ruminant production and the small ruminant genetic resource in tropical Africa, 1991 (E)
89 Manual for the production of Marek's disease, Gumboro disease and inactivated Newcastle disease vaccines, 1991 (E F)
90 Application of biotechnology to nutrition of animals in developing countries, 1991 (E F)
91 Guidelines for slaughtering, meat cutting and further processing, 1991 (E F)
92 Manual on meat cold store operation and management, 1991 (E S)
93 Utilization of renewable energy sources and energy-saving technologies by small-scale milk plants and collection centres, 1992 (E)
94 Proceedings of the FAO expert consultation on the genetic aspects of trypanotolerance, 1992 (E)
95 Roots, tubers, plantains and bananas in animal feeding, 1992 (E)
96 Distribution and impact of helminth diseases of livestock in developing countries, 1992 (E)
97 Construction and operation of medium-sized abattoirs in developing countries, 1992 (E)
98 Small-scale poultry processing, 1992 (Ar E)
99 *In situ* conservation of livestock and poultry, 1992 (E)
100 Programme for the control of African animal trypanosomiasis and related development, 1992 (E)
101 Genetic improvement of hair sheep in the tropics, 1992 (E)
102 Legume trees and other fodder trees as protein sources for livestock, 1992 (E)
103 Improving sheep reproduction in the Near East, 1992 (Ar)
104 The management of global animal genetic resources, 1992 (E)
105 Sustainable livestock production in the mountain agro-ecosystem of Nepal, 1992 (E)
106 Sustainable animal production from small farm systems in South-East Asia, 1993 (E)
107 Strategies for sustainable animal agriculture in developing countries, 1993 (E F)
108 Evaluation of breeds and crosses of domestic animals, 1993 (E)
109 Bovine spongiform encephalopathy, 1993 (Ar E)
110 L'amélioration génétique des bovins en Afrique de l'Ouest, 1993 (F)
111 L'utilización sostenible de hembras F1 en la producción del ganado lechero tropical, 1993 (S)
112 Physiologie de la reproduction des bovins trypanotolérants, 1993 (F)
113 La technologie des fromages au lait de dromadaire (*Camelus dromedarius*), 1993 (F)
114 Food losses due to non-infectious and production diseases in developing countries, 1993 (E)
115 Manuel de formation pratique pour la transplantation embryonnaire chez la brebis et la chèvre, 1993 (F S)
116 Quality control of veterinary vaccines in developing countries, 1993 (E)
117 L'hygiène dans l'industrie alimentaire, 1993 – Les produits et l'aplication de l'hygiène, 1993 (F)
118 Quality control testing of rinderpest cell culture vaccine, 1994 (E)
119 Manual on meat inspection for developing countries, 1994 (E)
120 Manual para la instalación del pequeño matadero modular de la FAO, 1994 (S)
121 A systematic approach to tsetse and trypanosomiasis control, 1994 (E/F)
122 El capibara (*Hydrochoerus hydrochaeris*) – Estado actual de su producción, 1994 (S)
123 Edible by-products of slaughter animals, 1995 (E S)
124 L'approvisionnement des villes africaines en lait et produits laitiers, 1995 (F)
125 Veterinary education, 1995 (E)
126 Tropical animal feeding – A manual for research workers, 1995 (E)
127 World livestock production systems – Current status, issues and trends, 1996 (E)
128 Quality control testing of contagious bovine pleuropneumonia live attenuated vaccine – Standard operating procedures, 1996 (E F)
129 The world without rinderpest, 1996 (E)
130 Manual de prácticas de manejo de alpacas y llamas, 1996 (S)
131 Les perspectives de développement de la filière lait de chèvre dans le bassin méditerranéen, 1996 (F)
132 Feeding pigs in the tropics, 1997 (E)
133 Prevention and control of transboundary animal diseases, 1997 (E)
134 Tratamiento y utilización de residuos de origen animal, pesquero y alimenticio en la alimentación animal, 1997 (S)
135 Roughage utilization in warm climates, 1997 (E F)
136 Proceedings of the first Internet Conference on Salivarian Trypanosomes, 1997 (E)
137 Developing national emergency prevention systems for transboundary animal diseases, 1997 (E)

138	Producción de cuyes (*Cavia porcellus*), 1997 (S)
139	Tree foliage in ruminant nutrition, 1997 (E)
140/1	Analisis de sistemas de producción animal – Tomo 1: Las bases conceptuales, 1997 (S)
140/2	Analisis de sistemas de producción animal – Tomo 2: Las herramientas basicas, 1997 (S)
141	Biological control of gastro-intestinal nematodes of ruminants using predacious fungi, 1998 (E)
142	Village chicken production systems in rural Africa – Household food security and gender issues,1998 (E)
142	Village chicken production systems in rural Africa – Household food security and gender issues,1998 (E)
143	Agroforestería para la producción animal en América Latina, 1999 (S)
144	New technologies in the fight against transboundary animal diseases, 1999 (E)

Availability: December 1999

Ar	–	Arabic	Multil	–	Multilingual
C	–	Chinese	*		Out of print
E	–	English	**		In preparation
F	–	French			
P	–	Portuguese			
S	–	Spanish			

The FAO Technical Papers are available through the authorized FAO Sales Agents or directly from Sales and Marketing Group, FAO, Viale delle Terme di Caracalla, 00100 Rome, Italy.